HOW CANCER

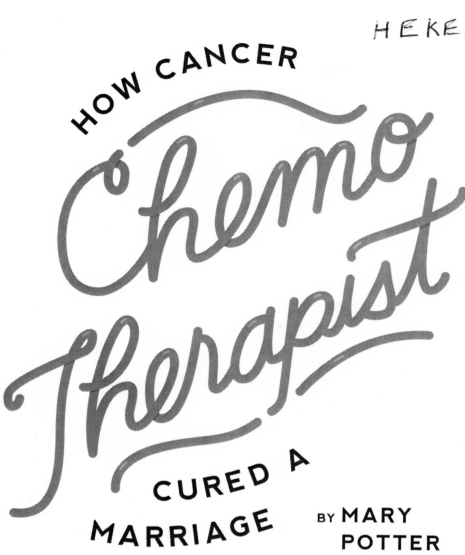

Chemo Therapist

CURED A
MARRIAGE

BY MARY
POTTER
KENYON

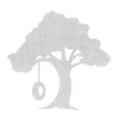

Published by Familius LLC, www.familius.com

Familius books are available at special discounts for bulk purchases for sales promotions, family or corporate use. Special editions, including personalized covers, excerpts of existing books, or books with corporate logos, can be created in large quantities for special needs. For more information, contact Premium Sales at 559-876-2170 or email specialmarkets@familius.com

Reproduction of this book in any manner, in whole or in part, without written permission of the publisher is prohibited.

Library of Congress Catalog-in-Publication Data

2013957919

pISBN 978-1-939629-09-8

eISBN 978-1-938301-66-7

Printed in the United States of America

Edited by Maggie Wickes

Cover design by David Miles

Book design by Brooke Jorden

10 9 8 7 6 5 4 3 2 1

First Edition

Praise for
Chemo-Therapist

"Mary Potter Kenyon brings transparency, honesty, humor, and hope to spouses and family members caring for loved ones with cancer. With deep insight, she shares that illness can unlock doors to deeper levels in our relationships and lead us to new discoveries about ourselves and others. *Chemo-Therapist* is a must-read book about living and loving for anyone who wants to discover how to find joy in each day."

> —Shelly Beach, Christy award-winning author of *Ambushed By Grace: Help & Hope on the Caregiving Journey* and *Precious Lord, Take My Hand: Meditations for Caregivers*

"Mary Potter Kenyon tells a beautiful love story, describing her life as a mother of eight home-schooled children, struggling with financial problems, and the trauma of her husband's fight against oral cancer. She serves up strong illustrative details covered with a double topping of honesty. No sugar coating here. If you've ever driven past a stranger's house and wondered what goes on behind closed doors, you'll want to open this book. But be fully warned! You'll have trouble putting it down."

> —Elaine Fantle Shimberg, author of *Blending Families* and co-author of *The Complete Single Father*

"This intensely personal book openly talks about the issues that families face when a spouse is facing serious cancer treatments. Mary's frank writing about the emotional problems they faced as a family and as a couple should be required reading for couples facing any life and death medical condition. Finding 'the gift' of a new relationship in the midst of stress and daily living will, I hope, inspire others to reach for the same goal."

—Jean Reed, co-author with her husband, Donn, of *Lifetime Learning Companion*

"Mary Potter Kenyon shares the story of what happened to her family when her husband David was diagnosed with oral cancer, and the story she weaves is compelling, enlightening, and utterly engaging. Every so often, a book comes along which seizes the reader's attention and draws him into the life and the everyday concerns of another person, a book which informs and illuminates and makes the reader stop and think hard about his own life. This is such a book."

—Helen Hegener, author of *Alternatives in Education*, *The Homeschool Reader*, and *The Mantanuska Colony Barns*

This book is dedicated to the husband who taught me what it is to truly love a spouse; the siblings who supported us during David's cancer journey; my friend Mary, who spent many hours editing the first draft of this manuscript; and the two women who helped me believe in myself and my story: Shelly Beach and Wanda Sanchez.

Foreword

In my work as a radiation oncologist, I spend a good deal of time preparing for my first official visit with my patients. To me, this visit will set the tone for what will eventually become a long-standing relationship. This relationship comes about because of an unwanted intruder (cancer) in a patient's life. This intruder takes many patients and their families on a roller coaster of emotions, disappointments, and expectations. I still remember the day I first met David and Mary Kenyon. I remember exactly where we were when I had to discuss with them a plan for an aggressive, multifaceted treatment for David that would most likely change the fabric of their lives forever. Little did I know then how much they would teach me.

My mentors at the University of California, Los Angeles School of Medicine (UCLA) instilled in me the dictum that a physician must always learn from the patient, for patients have so much to teach us, if we will only listen. I hope that you, the reader, will listen to the honest, heartfelt, and sometimes painfully difficult experiences of a family struggling to make sense of what the diagnosis of cancer meant to them. For those of you with a diagnosis of cancer in your family, reading this book will reinforce for you that you are not alone in trying to come to terms with your worries, your struggles, and your feelings. Reading this book will show you that you have an inner strength you never believed possible.

Mary Kenyon addresses important questions about how a spouse, children, relatives, and friends relate to this new intruder in their lives. Cancer does not have to change everything in a negative way. Remarkably, there are positives as well. Mary lived every day of her life during her husband's treatment looking for the positive while fighting to bring happiness and stability into her family's life. I believe she succeeded. You can, too.

For physicians, I hope this book shines a light on what happens to our patients and their families when they leave our offices after that first important visit. I believe that this book can become a powerful tool in educating your patients (and you!), which, in turn, can only serve to strengthen the physician/patient bond. Within that bond lies the potential for success.

David and Mary Kenyon have been a blessing in my life. I have no doubt that they will be a blessing in your life, too.

Susanna R. Gordon, MD
Diplomate, The American Board of Radiology

Contents

Introduction

If you have picked up this book, you may have been diagnosed with cancer, will be caring for someone through cancer treatment, or know someone who has cancer. Before you read any further, I want you to know that my husband *did not die* from his cancer. Instead, he became a five-year survivor in June 2011—a milestone year when the medical establishment labels those who have experienced cancer a "survivor."

Why do I feel the need to point this out? When my husband was diagnosed with cancer in June 2006, I immediately began searching for books about the disease, particularly those that had been written from the viewpoint of a caregiver. Unfortunately, the majority of them ended with the spouse dying, something I was not willing to consider. I refused to read those books. If it is indeed true that a cancer patient's outlook affects the eventual outcome, then why would anyone at the beginning of his or her cancer journey want to read about a cancer experience that ends in death?

If you get nothing more out of this true story of caregiving, my hope is that you will at least see how good can come from something as inherently bad as cancer, and how the act of caring for a spouse can dramatically improve a marriage relationship. There were many times in the years after his grueling cancer treatment that my husband would glance over at me appreciatively, take hold of my hand, and announce: "If it took cancer to get our marriage to this point, then I am glad for the cancer." If you are just starting down the path that David and I found ourselves on as a couple, I can assure you that, together, you can face whatever comes your way and come out on the other side of the experience stronger, closer, and—dare I say it? Yes—happier.

The majority of this manuscript was written during the months of my husband's cancer treatment in 2006. I began writing while he recovered in the hospital from the invasive surgery that removed his tumor. Sitting next to his hospital bed, I held his hand with one of mine while I wrote with the other. I continued writing every Wednesday while I kept him company in the room where he received weekly chemotherapy infusions. I rose early every morning before my children woke up so I could write some more. Writing became my therapy, a way of working through the myriad of emotions cancer and caregiving brought into my life. Initially, I didn't know I was writing a book. By the end of David's treatment, I realized I'd written the very book I had been searching for upon his diagnosis.

Is This All There Is?

Chapter One

Big families are like waterbed stores. They used to be everywhere; now they're just weird.

—Jim Gaffigan, comedian

I jerked the strap of the baby carrier higher up on my shoulder, adjusting the weight of eleven-month-old Abby against my back. Squinting with the sun's glare, my eyes searched the second floor windows of the brick building. Had anyone even noticed I'd left? An exasperated sigh escaped me as a small hand firmly grasped a fist full of the tender hairs at the base of my neck. I reflexively began walking with the surprisingly strong tugs, picking up my pace in the hope that the bouncing motion would lull Abby to sleep. Of all days, why had she chosen this one to skip a much-needed nap? Had she sensed our tenseness? She'd clung to me all morning, and my husband David's lame attempts to entertain her while I got dressed only seemed to aggravate the situation. The few words her father and I had exchanged that morning were terse ones, hissed out between clenched teeth. We'd timed the twenty-seven minute drive to coincide with Abby's naptime, and yet, even that had failed to pacify her. She'd cried all the way.

By the fourth round of circling the building, I was fuming, negative thoughts churning inside my head:

Why is Abby stubbornly refusing to fall asleep? Why do I always have to miss all the fun? It seems like at every single event in the last twenty-five years I am so busy caring for a baby or chasing a toddler, I am unable to properly visit with anyone. I've become the perpetual haggard mother, having spent a mind-boggling eighteen years either pregnant or nursing. I shook my head to clear it, and the movement startled Abby, who resumed crying. Beads of sweat dotted my forehead and upper lip, and my eyes welled with tears of frustration. *It's typical that I am walking alone outside tending to a fussy baby while a group of family and friends celebrate in a room above the bank. Was ours even a marriage to celebrate? Who has a baby at their twenty-fifth wedding anniversary party anyway?*

People like us—that's who. Most of our marriage had served as a prime example of living outside the box. Our unorthodox choices in having a large family, living off one income, homeschooling, and practicing an attachment-style parenting made us an anomaly among most of the couples we knew.

I met David in the summer of 1978; I was working as a waitress before beginning classes at the University of Northern Iowa that fall. He was already a student there, taking summer courses. He often stopped at the restaurant for a cup of coffee and to flirt with the waitresses, a pastime he vehemently denied later. I was extremely shy and uncomfortable in my own skin. Not only did I slosh coffee on him at our initial meeting, I did the same with iced tea or coffee on several of our first dates. It became a joke between us: my nervous habit of knocking over glasses of beverages.

I was smitten mostly by David's treatment of me as if I were a rare and precious find, his transparent admiration a boon to my fragile ego. We dated for four months before he asked me to marry him; it took another two before I said yes. We planned our own wedding: a simple affair that cost us less than $400, including the dress and rings. The one thing I never expected or desired from our marriage was wealth. I'd grown up in poverty, and both of us were aiming for degrees related to social work, so it was unlikely our future jobs would pay well. We enjoyed a naïve romanticism living as struggling college students.

We got married on a sunny June day in 1979, a few days before the summer classes began. Being raised a staunch Catholic, I couldn't morally rationalize using any artificial birth control and was only vaguely familiar with the concept of Natural Family Planning (NFP). Since I was well past the middle of my cycle, we assumed we were safe from pregnancy during our brief honeymoon at an inexpensive motel over the weekend. At the time, we would have been surprised to learn that the stress of planning a wedding could throw off a menstrual cycle. I likely conceived our first child on our wedding night because by the second week of classes, I was hit by waves of nausea so bad that I called David from work to bring me home and take care of me. He did so, tucking me into bed and ministering to my needs that day and for several more days, until my continued illness prompted a visit to the campus doctor. My new husband treated me with great tenderness when he discovered I was carrying his child. He developed "couvade syndrome" during my pregnancy, suffering with sympathetic symptoms of pregnancy: weight gain, heartburn, muscle aches, and leg cramps. At night, the baby vigorously kicked his back as we spooned in bed.

Those were the halcyon days of our marriage: living in married student housing, taking classes and working, and staggering our hours so that little Danny never had to have a babysitter. His early years were spent walking the sidewalks of the UNI campus. Danny's first word was "clock," due to the large clock tower on the grounds.

He accompanied us to our designated trade-off destinations, dragging a stuffed pink panther behind him. Occasionally, he attended classes with me—a suntanned, blonde-haired toddler sitting uncharacteristically quietly at a huge desk with his small tote bag of drawing materials and a snack.

We lived a sort of surreal existence, enjoying a mostly carefree lifestyle in the artificial and communal-like student housing and applying for loans and grants to supplement our work income. We would enter the financial aid office with detailed lists of the books we needed money for, only to be told by the loan officer that our financial package must cover what they estimated our living expenses to be as well. Their figures were always inflated as we lived very simply. We'd walk out with a check large enough to cover textbooks along with our one splurge: the local Happy Chef restaurant's 99-cent breakfast. Danny spent many hours sitting in that restaurant, sliding melting ice cubes back and forth across the shiny surface of the metal highchair while David and I held hands, talked, and drank gallons of coffee.

Our second child, a daughter we named Elizabeth, or Beth, after our two grandmothers, was born two and a half years after Danny. We continued our tag-team parenting for many more years and two more children, even after we'd both earned a Bachelor's degree and began taking graduate courses. David was taking classes at the University of Iowa when I gave birth to our third, a son named Michael Byron, the Byron for my father who had died during my pregnancy. It was a year later, after we had moved back to Cedar Falls where I'd begun graduate courses in Family Services, when I got pregnant with our fourth. I took my last finals from my hospital bed the day after I'd given birth to Rachel. By then, David was employed as a social worker in a small town an hour away. When we moved closer to his job, it was the first time in ten years of marriage that neither of us was attending classes somewhere.

Living in the real world came as quite a shock to us. Not only was there no financial aid office to help us out, but living on one income and being required to begin paying back all the money that office had so lavishly extended to us made the budget pretty tight. I scoured thrift shops to clothe our ever-expanding family and became a coupon queen at our local grocery store. Still, in the day-to-day struggle of paying bills and caring for little children, we quickly lost that naïve romanticism that had blessed our marriage in the college years. By 1991, we'd settled into a routine: David employed in social work, our two older children attending school, and me staying at home with our two youngest, except for the occasional evening when I left to attend a town council or school board meeting. I'd begun selling articles I'd written and was working part-time for a local newspaper covering occasional meetings and writing a biweekly column on parenting. It was around this time that a crisis in our lives arrived in the form of a chronic illness.

The day after Thanksgiving 1991, I woke up with what I thought was the stomach flu. I spent most of that day in the bathroom. While I still felt weak and shaky for the next few days, I just assumed it was from the illness or fatigue from having hosted a family get-together. The younger kids were used to me taking them for daily walks, and I assured them we'd get back to walking when Mommy got better.

Only Mommy didn't get better. The extreme fatigue, nausea, fever, sore muscles, and severe stomach upsets continued for days, then weeks. What began as a visit to the doctor to find out what was wrong with me became a three-month odyssey to specialists who ordered dozens of tests that all came back negative.

David watched helplessly as his wife's once robust health took a downward spiral. He started taking off work to accompany me to

7

appointments. At one point I started to wonder if the doctors were right and the illness was all in my head, but David knew better and convinced me to keep searching for answers.

Each morning, David set up bowls of cereal in front of the television for five-year-old Michael and three-year-old Rachel while I disappeared into the bathroom. At noon, he'd call to see if I was alright. A good day meant I was in the bathroom only half the morning. On particularly bad days, Dan would stay home from school and entertain his siblings.

In the middle of the night, Rachel would wake up looking for me. She knew to find me in the bathroom and would lay facedown on the floor, waiting for me to finish being sick. I lost thirty-five pounds on a diet of 7-Up and toast, becoming increasingly weaker. I distinctly remember the day I was outside hanging wet towels on the clothesline when I saw a recipe card, which must have fallen from my counter into the laundry basket, fly out with a gust of wind. I stood and watched it skip with the breeze through the grass and towards the ditch. I didn't even have the energy to chase after the favorite carrot cake recipe.

I was finally diagnosed with Chronic Fatigue Syndrome (CFS) in the spring of 1992, by a doctor my mother had introduced me to— one who was willing to consider the possibility that I was ill with something for which there was no medical test. He prescribed medication for the severe bouts of irritable bowel that had ruled my days.

Once I had a name for what ailed me and a drug to control the worst symptom, I learned to live with a chronic illness. I knew that one day of activity might mean three days of recovery, so I planned accordingly. I also immersed myself in literature about CFS, learning everything I could about it in those pre-Internet days. I made several trips back to Cedar Falls and the college library, looking for answers to what had triggered my illness and what could be done about it. I uncovered studies that attempted to link immune system disorders such as CFS, Epstein Barr, Parkinson's, and MS to certain immunizations. One article even suggested that caregivers of children who had recently had the MMR shot were exposing themselves to a trigger for an immune system disorder when they had close contact with the child's bodily fluids and feces. While I thought that somewhat far-fetched, the theory did make me search for Rachel's immunization records, where I discovered that she'd gotten her MMR shot the month I became ill. I couldn't have had much closer contact with her; she shared our bed and nursed frequently during the night.

By this time, in response to a pen-pal ad I'd run in a *Women's Circle* magazine, I was corresponding with other women who had CFS. One of them confided to me that she wished she could get pregnant, as she personally knew two women who had improved during a pregnancy. I couldn't unearth any research to back this claim up, but by the fall of 1992, I was sick and tired of being sick and tired, and I prayed that I would get pregnant if it would help me get better. By the following spring, I was indeed pregnant with our fifth child. I fretted and worried during the first trimester as morning sickness mimicked the worst of my illness, but by the beginning of the middle trimester, I felt amazing. For the first time in two years, I had my old energy back. It was during this pregnancy I decided to homeschool, something that had intrigued me ever since I'd interviewed a homeschooling couple for the newspaper the year before. I was relieved to remove Michael from school since his once sunny disposition had dramatically changed as soon as he began Junior Kindergarten. Elizabeth chose to be homeschooled as well. David and I thought we had probably gotten through the most stressful time of our marriage.

We were wrong.

I was actually looking forward to giving birth again. Unlike my first two births that had taken place in a teaching hospital where I was shaved, given an enema, hooked up to an IV, and relegated to laboring in a bed, my third and fourth births had been uneventful and extremely satisfying in terms of feeling empowered. I'd walked the hallways for most of my labor both times, stopping only long enough to push the babies out.

When I reached the hospital for my fifth delivery at six centimeters dilated, both the doctor and I expected things to go the same as they had with my previous two. I walked the hallway with my husband for a couple of hours, leaning against him or the wall whenever the contractions came. Suddenly, though, I doubled over with a different kind of pain, coming in constant waves without a break; I couldn't continue walking. I grabbed a phone off the wall and called my mother, who was watching the other children.

"Please pray. Something is wrong," I managed to gasp out before a nurse in the hallway hurried over and helped me back to the bed. Her face went white when she glanced down, and she ran out of the room.

Instinctively, I knew my baby was in trouble, so I wasn't surprised when my doctor hurried in, accompanied by several nurses. They immediately began prepping me for an emergency cesarean. As the doctor explained that the bleeding and pain I was experiencing signaled a sign of trouble, he handed my husband a form to sign, giving permission for the surgery. With no surgeon on staff, I was lucky there was one visiting his patient down the hall. I felt the first slice of the scalpel as I was being put under general anesthesia. The next thing I knew, I woke up to see my husband holding our son, Matthew. I'd experienced placenta previa, when the placenta pulls away from the uterus and threatens to emerge before the baby. This medical emergency left the doctor shaking his head and informing

David privately that it was the closest he'd ever come to losing both mother and baby. I'd lost so much blood and was so weak and anemic that I required a blood transfusion and an extended hospital stay. When I arrived home, David took off an extra week from his job to care for me and our new son. The day he returned to work, he was unexpectedly fired.

To describe those following weeks as stressful is an understatement. Unlike my recovery from previous births, I didn't bounce back from the emergency surgery. David not only had to deal with the loss of a job, he was thrust into the position of caring for an ailing wife. Within weeks of Matthew's birth, and before I had fully recovered, I signed a contract with a publisher for a book on how to save money in homeschooling. Because of my commitment to a deadline, David spent an inordinate amount of time caring for our newborn. If that weren't emasculating enough, it seemed as though every single social work job he applied for went to a woman. I watched my husband get more and more depressed as he applied for dozens of jobs. Those months of unemployment became the second most difficult period of our marriage, but by no means our biggest trial.

That would come three more daughters and thirteen years later, in June 2006, the month my husband David was diagnosed with cancer.

Diagnosis: Cancer

Chapter Two

A strong, positive mental attitude will create more miracles than any wonder drug.

—Patricia Neal

For years, my rare, lone bubble baths included at least one floating toy army man or hard plastic cow figure, and usually by bath's end, an ecstatic toddler who'd stripped off his or her clothes and jumped in. The end tables in our home were inevitably strewn with books and toys, and our van was littered with candy wrappers and stray shoes. Small fingerprints marred our woodwork and windows. Ours was a child-centered home, which just made sense, since the children outnumbered adults ever since 1987.

By 2006, we were living in rural Dyersville, Iowa, in a rented farmhouse with our five youngest children. Unable to find a job in his chosen profession of social work, David had been working in maintenance at a nursing home for almost nine years while I stayed home and homeschooled our children. My job was to stretch our limited income as far as possible, and I'd gotten quite proficient at it, matching sale prices with coupons and stockpiling items that were either free or cost just pennies. I dressed our children well with

13

bargains from the clearance racks and thrift store finds. A couple of our babies were outfitted completely in high-end boutique quality organic cotton children's clothing, courtesy of a woman who bartered with me, sending me gently used, expensive infant clothing in exchange for books I found for her. I supplemented our income by selling short articles and essays I wrote. I'd also spent several years selling extra books from our family book sale hunts, paying for our own purchases in the process and networking with other homeschoolers. I was busy all the time, and if asked, would have said that was typical for any homeschooling mother of a large family. I can think of many mornings when, in the daze of a long to-do list, I actually encouraged my husband David to leave for work so we could begin our real day without him. Many times he left with little more than a perfunctory peck on the cheek from me.

David and I hadn't exactly lost sight of our marriage, but it had been a long time since we'd held hands, drank gallons of coffee like we had while in college, or just spent time alone talking. We'd gotten apathetic when it came to working at our relationship, and I had accepted it as a natural state for a couple busy with small children. David had been sleeping on a mattress on the floor of our bedroom for almost three years, since the birth of our youngest, Abby, in July 2003. It was just easier for nighttime nursing to share a bed with my last three babies. With each baby, it seemed to take longer to ease them into their own bed. Emily was born in 1996 and slept with us for over two years. Katie was born in January 2000 and stayed in our room until her sister was born in 2003.

A week before her third birthday, I decided it was high time to wean Abby to a toddler bed. That same week, David visited an ear, nose, and throat specialist (ENT) about a lump he'd noticed on the left side of his neck. Our doctor had already prescribed a dose of antibiotics to see if his lymph nodes were swollen from a virus.

When the lump got bigger, he ordered a CT scan, which showed a definite mass on the left side of David's neck. I'm not sure what I expected to learn when I went to the appointment with David, but I certainly wasn't prepared to hear the "C" word.

It took Dr. Alt, the ENT, only a few minutes to find a growth on the far back side of David's tongue. As he explained that he'd found a suspicious growth on the tongue and he needed to do a biopsy of the swollen lymph nodes, it dawned on me what he wasn't saying.

"Are you talking about cancer?" I asked, hoping he would say no.

"Yes," he said. "It looks like cancer."

At that moment, it seemed an abrupt and jarring answer, but later, we would come to appreciate Dr. Alt's forthrightness and professionalism. After all, was there a better way to inform a patient of bad news? I guessed that Dr. Alt let the personality of his patients dictate his response. I asked, and he truthfully answered. As much as I wanted to hear him say it wasn't cancer, he knew it probably was, and it wouldn't have done us any good to pretend otherwise.

David and I were quiet after this pronouncement, absorbing the shock. David had smoked for several years as a teen, but had quit thirty-five years before. When he said this, Dr. Alt explained that even nonsmokers get oral cancer, and it didn't really matter why David had gotten it; what mattered was how to treat it.

After doing a needle biopsy of the lymph nodes, Dr. Alt sat down on a rolling stool, pushing it close to David so he was eye-level with him. Looking directly into my husband's eyes, he slowly and succinctly explained what David could expect. I listened closely, wondering just how much my husband actually heard after the word *cancer*. According to Dr. Alt, David needed surgery to remove the tumor and the portion of the tongue around it, along with removal of the affected lymph nodes. Because the tongue would swell, a tracheotomy and a breathing tube would be necessary, along with a feeding tube, since he would be unable to eat. Since the cancer had obviously spread to the lymph nodes, it was assumed David would be needing radiation treatments after he recovered from surgery. After this explanation, Dr. Alt leaned back, waiting for our questions. Seeing our stricken faces, he stressed then that this was not a death sentence and that the cancer would very likely be removed through surgery and radiation treatment. "People can live for years after this type of cancer," he assured us.

When we left the office that day, we were shell-shocked, hit with so much information in so little time. Clutching each other's hands, we were very quiet all the way back to Dyersville. I glanced over at my husband at the wheel, making the conscious decision right then to be there for him no matter what came our way. We stopped at our son Dan's shop where he worked on custom-designed t-shirts. As I stepped through the door and saw Dan's concerned face, I burst into tears.

All of a sudden, it was real. David had cancer.

We called our married daughter Elizabeth from Dan's shop to break the news to her. She was as stunned as Dan had been. When we arrived home, we had to tell the younger children. Because we homeschooled and our children were around me all day, every day, they were experts at picking up on every little emotional nuance. There was no way we could hide something this big from them. Matthew (12) and Emily (10) asked the most questions, probably because they knew enough about cancer to be frightened, but not enough to feel reassured that their dad could be cured. Sobered by the news, Rachel (17) and Michael (19) were quietly supportive through their actions around the house in the next few days: Rachel chipped in with household chores I normally had to beg her to do, and Michael went out of his way to keep his younger siblings entertained whenever he was around.

As soon as I could extract myself from the children's apprehensive clinging, I logged onto the computer to tell my extended family members, partly so they could start praying, but mostly for emotional support. I grew up in a large family, and most of my siblings remained very close-knit. I badly needed a virtual hug from them, so I posted on our family's web page:

> *Some of you know David had a lump on the side of his neck. I went to the specialist with him today in Dubuque, and he has a tumor on the back of his tongue and growth in the lymph nodes on that side, too. The doctor says it does look like cancer. He did a biopsy, and we will know the results of that later, but he didn't seem to have any doubts what it was. Please pray for us as I don't know what I would do without David. As it is, he will have to have surgery to remove the tumor, and he won't be able to breathe on his own, eat, or talk for a while afterwards, so he will have a tracheotomy and a feeding tube. Please pray for him.*

Writing about it brought fresh waves of fear and sadness. Almost as a postscript, I added:

> *Hug your spouse tonight.*

I then called my mother, who knew we'd gone to see a specialist that day and was waiting for an update. When I filled her in on the news, she gasped in dismay and told me she would be praying. I knew her rosary would come out as soon as she got off the phone and that she'd want to talk to other family members in between the clacking of the beads. At her advancing age, my mother was unable to do much more for us than pray, but I had no doubt thousands of her prayers were directed heavenward for us in the coming months.

"Let me be the one to call Jane," I requested before hanging up.

The hardest person to tell was my youngest sister, Jane, mostly because she was going through a health crisis of her own, but also because she had always been there for me, and now she was so far away in Washington. Even though Jane had lived in Texas when I'd had CFS, she had called me regularly, never once doubting me or my illness. If it hadn't been for her emotional support, I don't know what I would have done. Her phone calls, as well as my mother's, had been a lifeline for me then, and I needed that lifeline now. I hesitated briefly before dialing her number. Jane was facing a second cross-country move in less than a month, and dealing with a serious bout with an undiagnosed physical disorder that caused extreme flushing and pain in her face and extremities. She'd suffered with it for several years, but the pain had gotten so severe that now she'd resorted to spending most of her day sitting in front of a fan, barely moving—unable to do housework, go to stores, speak on the phone for any length of time, or even use the computer. She had become a prisoner in her own home. There wasn't anything she could do about it except hope that the specialist she was scheduled to see at the Mayo Clinic in a couple of months would be able to help. My brother-in-law Philip answered the phone but quickly handed it to Jane when he heard my shaking voice.

"What is it? Is it Mom?" Jane asked when I started sobbing into the phone.

"No," I managed to get out, before weeping again. I knew one of Jane's greatest fears was that something would happen to our mother when she was so far away.

"Are you OK? The kids?" she asked again.

"It's David. He has cancer," I blurted out before starting to cry uncontrollably again.

It had become almost a joke between us—how talking to her on the phone inevitably made me tear up. Either she was just a good listener, or maybe it was because when I needed her the most she was always so far away.

There was an audible gasp before the phone went quiet. Gathering my emotions, I continued, "It's a tumor on his tongue that spread to his lymph nodes. He'll need surgery and radiation." I went into more detail about how invasive the surgery would be and how long recovery would take.

Then my dear sister, who had always listened to me cry and whine, and who had never broken down when discussing her own illness and the pain she suffered from it, began crying, too.

"Oh, Mary, I'm so sorry," she said. "We love you both so much. I am so sorry you are going through this. We love you and will be praying for both of you."

Our phone call ended with her dismissing my belated inquiries about her own health. We both left unsaid what she meant: David's health concern could end in death, while hers likely would not.

Telling David's family was easier, if only because they lived so far away and we saw them so rarely. Like me, David had grown up in a large family, but after leaving the area and getting married, he often felt somewhat detached from their lives. That didn't mean he didn't love his siblings or that they didn't love him. But his life seemed so far removed from theirs. A prime example of this familial distance, he hadn't found out his mother was in a nursing home until days after the fact. Only David's brother Keith had met our youngest child, Abby. There were two siblings we hadn't even seen for six years, and only then because we'd traveled three hours in sub-zero weather in an old van crammed full of children to join them for their annual Christmas Eve get-together. This kind of emotional and physical distance among siblings was unfathomable to me, but something I had recognized in his family from early on in our dating days.

The reasons for their familial relationship may have been partly due to their parents' divorce, but I was fairly certain it had more to do with the fact that, as my fiancé, David had to pull his father out of a tavern each time we visited him. His mother couldn't have had an easy time of it raising her youngest children alone after her husband left his first family to start another one with a woman the same age as his oldest daughter. Whatever the reasons for a strained family relationship, I'd made an attempt to keep in touch with his siblings, and in recent years most of them had responded by remembering our children's birthdays and sending cards on David's. David felt an especially close bond with his brother Keith, so I called him the night of the diagnosis. I left a message on their answering machine, and when Keith called back later, I briefly explained the diagnosis before handing the phone over to David. I had no inkling then that Keith would become a huge phone support for me during David's hospitalization.

Those first days after the diagnosis were extremely difficult for me. When David was home from work, I put on my supportive, optimistic façade. While he was gone, I could think about very little except his cancer. Yet, I was supposed to continue operating our busy household as before, running errands in town and caring for increasingly needy children who were also worried about their dad.

I was an emotional wreck, crying at the slightest provocation. Running errands the morning after David's diagnosis, the bank teller at the drive-up asked how I was doing, and I couldn't answer past the lump in my throat. Tears blurred my vision as I hurriedly drove away.

Later that same day, with David still at work, I began sobbing again as I stood at the clothesline, folding his t-shirts as I took them down. The little girls saw me crying and ran over to hug me, begging me to stop. Dan and Elizabeth must've felt as bereft as I did, because

Elizabeth called and asked me to visit, and Dan stopped to see me just as I was headed out the door to go see Elizabeth.

When I started crying again, he snapped, "Stop it, Mom. You're acting like Dad is going to die."

I realized with horror that he was right. Dan and I both ended up at Elizabeth's house the rest of the afternoon, taking great comfort in each other's presence, and discussing the things we had each discovered about cancer in our respective Internet searches the night before.

Unlike my rudimentary library searches for CFS information years before, the Internet provided hundreds of informational cancer sites to choose from within the confines of our homes. We learned more about cancer than we had ever wanted to know. We were surprised to discover that cancer is the second leading cause of death in the United States and that half of all men and one third of all women in the United States would develop some form of it in their lifetime. We'd heard of people with cancer, but out of our large families and extended families had personally known only one: a nephew who had survived a brain tumor several years before. Later, we would discover that David's oldest sister was a five-year survivor of uterine cancer, but at the time of David's diagnosis, we hadn't known that. The stark cancer statistics frightened us. Before, cancer seemed like something that happened to other people. Suddenly we realized it could happen to any one of us, and the odds were that it would happen again in our family.

Among all the facts and figures on cancer, one statistic stood out from all the rest: a good support system seemed crucial in the survival rates of cancer patients. After reading half a dozen reports reiterating this fact, I was ready to build up the best support team I could for David and myself, and determined to be the best darn caregiver I could be. The problem was, I didn't know anyone else who had navigated the world of cancer with their spouse. Then I remembered Jean Reed.

Jean was one of the few people I knew whose spouse had gone through treatment for cancer. Her husband, Donn, had written the first-ever book for homeschoolers that reviewed products and resources, *The Home School Source Book*. He had sent me a personal note of encouragement when I was doing research for my own homeschooling book. Later, I was shocked to hear he'd died of cancer and intrigued to find out that Jean was completing a new edition of his book in his memory. At that time, I'd written her with my condolences and told her about the note Donn had sent and how much it had meant to me as a fledgling writer. We'd struck up a correspondence of sorts, occasionally writing and usually sending Christmas cards, but I hadn't communicated with her in months.

Now it seemed important to get in touch with her again. Somehow I figured a woman whose husband had caught their four babies in his hands during home births would understand how scared I was for David. She, too, had watched the person she loved fight cancer. I briefly shared David's diagnosis with her in an e-mail message.

Her return e-mail was swift and sympathetic. Like the websites I'd perused, Jean reiterated how important a support system was for both David and me. Several days later, she sent a card, reminding me to take care of myself. I was surprised, but pleased, to get a phone call from her a few nights later. Jean knew firsthand what I was going through as a spouse of someone with cancer. After talking for several minutes, she mentioned going to her daughter's wedding and how glad she was that her recovery from surgery was going so well.

Surgery? It was only then she told me that she'd been diagnosed with breast cancer and had undergone a complete mastectomy!

There she was, comforting and supporting me, without sharing that she was fighting her own battle with cancer. While I'd already admired her, I came away from that phone call with a renewed appreciation for her strength and kindness, along with an awareness of how helpful it is to be able to talk to someone who'd gone down this path before us.

Those first few nights after the appointment with Dr. Alt, I was so grateful I'd moved Abby into her own bed. I couldn't fall asleep without having David next to me, and I clung to his hand through most of the night. I wondered how the gulf between us had gotten so big that I hadn't even missed him being next to me in bed the past few years. That first weekend after the diagnosis, we lay down on the bed together several times throughout the day—David holding me close, or sometimes, me holding him with his head on my chest. We took the time to just listen to each other's hearts—literally and figuratively. I realized how busy I'd always been with the house and the children, and how I'd neglected my relationship with David. I vowed not to let that happen again. Dan, Elizabeth, and I also began saying "I love you" on the phone to each other, something we rarely had done before. Even the little ones would dash through a room shouting, "I love you, Mom. I love you, Dad," in their wake. The realization that our whole world could change in an instant and that we could lose someone we loved shook us to the core.

We had become a kinder, gentler household.

Chapter Three

Cut It Out

If children have the ability to ignore all odds and percentages, then maybe we can all learn from them. When you think about it, what other choice is there but to hope? We have two options, medically and emotionally: give up, or fight like hell.

—Lance Armstrong

The official diagnosis of cancer was given over the phone several days later. When a nurse called to give us the results of the biopsy, she cautiously asked what Dr. Alt had told us. I said that he'd warned us it was probably cancer.

"Yes, it is cancer," she replied, and even though I'd expected it, my stomach lurched.

She said the next step would be to schedule a PET scan to see if there was cancer anywhere else in David's body. *Anywhere else?* We hadn't even imagined that possibility. Initially, the scan was scheduled for late in the day on July 3, and the results would be available the following day. After I hung up, I realized that the next day would be a holiday and we'd have to wait an additional day for results. I couldn't imagine waiting that extra day. I wanted to know as soon as possible if we were dealing with more cancer than the oral cancer and lymph node involvement. I briefly wondered what it would feel like if we discovered David's body was riddled with cancer. I shuddered at the thought. I called the nurse back and asked if we could get the results the same day if we were able to get a morning appointment. She said she would talk to the doctor and call me back.

My heart heavy, I went upstairs to tell David the results of the biopsy. I knew he had been holding onto the remote possibility that the biopsy would be negative. Not only did he indeed have cancer, but we hadn't even considered that it could have spread farther than the lymph nodes. How could we endure waiting forty-eight hours after the test to get the results? We were both surprised and relieved when the nurse called back and said David could have the PET scan early in the morning; Dr. Alt was scheduled for surgery all afternoon but would meet us afterwards at his office, specifically to give us the results. I knew how busy he must be. The initial good feeling I'd had about him was immediately reinforced.

Dan took David to the PET scan early in the morning, and I made the return trip to Dubuque with David that afternoon to meet with Dr. Alt for the results. The news was encouraging. It didn't look like the cancer had spread beyond the head and neck area. Dr. Alt and his colleague Dr. King both recommended surgery to remove the tumor on the tongue and the lymph nodes, followed by radiation. Dr. Alt did a biopsy of the tumor, just to make sure that it was the same kind of cancer as in the lymph nodes (squamous cell carcinoma), and told us thst after the results of that biopsy came back, the surgery would be scheduled.

Oddly enough, at this point, no one had given us a prognosis or statistics for the kind of cancer David had, and David hadn't asked. Dan, Elizabeth, and I had seen the sobering statistics in our

respective online searches. Several websites quoted a five-year survival rate of 50 percent for patients with oral cancer. Others gave
less optimistic results. Oral cancer also had a high recurrence rate.
Unless David specifically asked, we saw no reason to share those
statistics. While I worried about the numbers, Dan pointed out
that those statistics included the elderly, patients who smoked, and
those with compromised immune systems. In other words, the statistics meant very little for David's individual case. My two adult
children and I had read the same reports: a positive attitude and a
good support system seemed to be a crucial characteristic of cancer
survivors. We were going to do everything in our power to see that
David had both.

As expected, several days later, the results of the biopsy con-
firmed Dr. Alt's suspicion that the tumor on the tongue was the
origin of the cancer and it had spread to the lymph nodes. Surgery
was scheduled for the afternoon of July 12. We were to be at the
hospital by noon.

David and I didn't get much sleep the night before surgery. We
tossed and turned, occasionally reaching out to touch each other's
hands. I'd gotten used to reaching out to touch David throughout
the night.

As I watched the nurses prepare my husband for surgery, I
thought about how different it was on the other side of the gown.
In all the years of our marriage, it had always been me having the
surgery: the emergency c-section with our fifth child, a knee surgery,
then two more c-sections with our seventh and eighth. I could
finally see how powerless David must have felt seeing his spouse in a
hospital gown, hooked up to an IV. It was an experience I could have
done without. I held David's hand tightly while we tried to make
small talk. As the surgical nurse wheeled him away, we both said, "I

love you" one more time. I had a hard time keeping my emotions in check as I returned to the waiting room.

When my two older sisters, Denise and Pat, had offered to sit with me during David's surgery, I hadn't thought it would be necessary, but as I headed back to the waiting room, I was glad they would be there because I realized I didn't want to be alone at a time like this. When I got back to the waiting area, though, they hadn't yet arrived. Just as I lost my composure and felt hot tears streaking down my cheeks, I saw them getting off the elevator. They rushed over, worriedly asking what happened.

"Nothing," I answered a bit sheepishly. "They just took David away and you weren't here so I was all alone."

They hugged me, smiling sympathetically.

The afternoon was long, but made much shorter by my sisters' presence. The surgical team called occasionally to update me, so I didn't want to leave the waiting room. By evening, another sister, Joan, had joined us. We took turns answering the phone since the volunteer had long since disappeared.

Around 6:30 p.m., a nurse came in to take us to a private meeting room to discuss the surgery with Dr. Alt. He told us the surgery had gone well and that he was confident he'd gotten the entire cancerous tumor on the tongue. Then he voiced his concern about how big some of the thirty-two lymph nodes that he removed were, especially one in particular, which he feared might have some extracapsular extension, a term I wasn't familiar with. He added that we wouldn't have pathology reports on the lymph nodes for another five to six days, so right now we should just concentrate on David's recovery. After he left the room, my sister Joan, a nurse, commented that "extracapsular extension" meant the cancer may have escaped the lymph nodes and that David might need chemotherapy along with the radiation we'd already expected as part of the treatment.

I didn't want to hear that; in our first appointment with him, Dr. Alt had discussed how harsh chemotherapy was. All four of us then headed to the Intensive Care Unit (ICU) waiting room to wait for David's arrival from the surgical recovery room.

It was close to 9:00 p.m. before he arrived. A nurse said we could go back and see him in pairs for a few minutes. My sister Joan tried to prepare me for what I would see by telling me how pale David would be and how he would be hooked up to tubes and machines. As a nurse, I'm sure she had often seen patients in bad shape, but there was nothing she could have said that would've prepared the rest of us for what we saw as we entered the Intensive Care room.

David lay in the bed motionless, staples up most of the side of his neck and partway across, a drainage tube and bag coming out the side, a breathing tube from a hole in his neck, and an IV and wires hooked up to his arm. Eyes closed, he looked like he was dead. I swallowed once, afraid to touch him.

Just then, he slowly opened his eyes, groggily looking at me. After he gave a thumbs-up signal, I took his hand, immensely relieved. I knew what he meant: he'd gotten through the surgery and was alright. I clutched his hand as my three sisters took their turns to see him. Joan came in first and commented how good he looked for having just been through surgery, then Pat stepped in for a few moments; from the look on her face, I knew she was as shocked as I was. By the time Denise came in, I was feeling lightheaded and realized it had been a mistake to skip two meals that day. I was dizzy and seeing spots in front of my eyes, but didn't want to let go of David's hand. Denise took one look at my white face and whispered, "Let me hold his hand. You sit down."

We exchanged hands quickly. Since there were no chairs in the room, I crouched to the floor with my head down until the dizziness passed. When I got up and took his hand again, David opened his eyes and this time I saw something more: a pleading look.

"Are you in pain?" I asked, and he nodded.

"A lot of pain?" He nodded again.

"I'll get help," I said as I rushed out of the room. I had promised him before the surgery I'd be his advocate.

I grabbed a nurse by her arm, pulling her toward the room, asking, "Can you do something? He's in pain."

As she returned to the room with me, she quietly explained that since the surgery, he'd only had one dose of morphine.

"Don't worry," she said to both of us when David opened his eyes. "We'll get on top of the pain. We'll push your morphine button every ten minutes until you can do it for yourself," she assured us as she pushed the button. David closed his eyes again. Patting his arm, I told him to rest and that I would come back the next day to see him. His eyes remained closed as he slowly nodded.

Ashamed of my weakness, I still couldn't get out of that room fast enough. I was desperate to escape the sight of David in pain. My chest heaving with sobs, I slowly walked back to the waiting room. The hallway seemed miles long, and my feet felt like lead weights. It was all I could do to put one foot in front of the other. When I finally reached my sisters, they hugged me close, their own eyes wet with tears.

I don't remember much of the trip home that night. I drove on autopilot, not really seeing the road ahead of me. Instead, I saw my husband's pain-filled eyes. Dan met me at the door of the house and hugged me, not commenting on my red-rimmed eyes or disheveled appearance. I'd already explained his Dad's condition on the way home, using the cell phone Pat had given me. The children gathered around me, asking questions about their daddy, but I avoided saying anything about his pain level or how he looked. They were tired, so I took them upstairs and let the three little girls fall asleep on my bed. When I came back down, I asked Dan if he would go with me the next day to the hospital. Originally, we'd planned on staggering our visits, but I knew I couldn't face seeing David alone the next day if the pain hadn't abated. Not eager to face seeing his Dad's pain alone either, he readily agreed to accompany me.

I went to bed as soon as Dan left and slept a few hours before waking up with a start and checking the clock. It was 3:00 a.m., and I couldn't help but wonder if David was asleep or awake and if they'd gotten his pain managed yet. I went downstairs and called the ICU, and the nurse on duty told me he was sleeping and they'd increased the medication. I attempted to go back to sleep myself, but I missed David so much and couldn't stand the thought of his pain being so strong that they'd had to increase his medication. I ached with loneliness for him. I hated not being there with him, and yet I didn't know how I could stand to be there and not be able to do anything to help. I tossed and turned, wondering how the nurses would know anything about my husband when he couldn't talk. Would they treat him as just another name on a chart? I didn't think I could stand that.

As tired as I was, I couldn't sleep. Jumbled thoughts kept going through my head. How could I be David's advocate if I wasn't there? How would the nurses get to know him as a person if he couldn't talk? Then it suddenly came to me. I knew what I had to do: I needed to write a letter to the nurses to be inserted in his chart so that every new nurse who came on duty could read about him and would think of him as the special person he was and not just another medical case.

I got out of bed and went downstairs. In the dark, I sat in front of the computer and wrote:

To the nurses who are caring for my husband, David Kenyon:

Since he is unable to communicate right now, I am writing this so you can get to know the patient you are caring for who has been my husband and best friend for twenty-seven years. I truly believe that nurses are "angels in disguise" for choosing a career that involves caring for the ill and infirm, and my prayers and gratitude are with you while you care for my dear husband.

David is the proud father of eight wonderful children. If he could talk, he would tell you stories of them and their unique artistic gifts and abilities. His coworkers tell me that he is always bragging about his family, and I believe it. He was the first to hold each of our babies after birth and announce in awe, "I love this baby," as if surprised that, once again, his heart expanded to include another little person in our lives. It took eight babies to get his brown eyes that I love, and that little girl, Abby, is three years old now. The first words out of her mouth every morning are, "Where is my Daddy?" David also has two beautiful grandchildren and a son-in-law he is proud of.

David is the kind of man who gets up every morning and makes his wife a cup of tea to start the day. He'll do dishes without complaint, and though he never cooks, he also never complains about what is served at the table—even during the early days of my pregnancies when too often that has been a bowl of cold cereal with fruit on it.

David has always been protective of older people, rushing to help the proverbial old lady crossing the street.

He works in a nursing home in maintenance, but I know many residents there stop him in the hallway so he can listen to their stories, because he does. He really listens. In fact, David rushes to the aid of anyone who needs it, even having the endearing, yet annoying, habit of cleaning up the table and stacking dishes for the waitress at a restaurant, hoping to make her job a little easier, but inevitably unwittingly annoying her in the process. In a world where rudeness prevails, David still opens doors for others, even going out of his way to do so.

I want you to know these things about David so that each time you go into his room you will see the loving father of eight and the caring husband that I see each time I look at him. He is the daddy who takes his family to Chuck E. Cheese's once a year and poses in the photo booth with his wife for our annual picture-taking. We laugh and joke that we should put the Chuck E. Cheese's photo in our local newspaper for our anniversaries because that is what our marriage has been all about: sharing simple things and being there for each other. If he could now, he would be telling you corny jokes and storing in his head those he hears back to share with his brothers who have the same dorky sense of humor.

So, dear nurses, please care for this special person as if he were your own father, your own brother, your own husband, because I can't bear to think of him in pain or feeling lonely, and I can't be there with him every minute of the day like I wish I could. Thank you so much for your loving care and for choosing this noble profession.

I pushed the print button on my computer, made a couple copies, and put them in my purse. Then I went back upstairs and finally fell asleep, just an hour before Abby woke up.

Chapter Four

Where Is My Daddy?

To the world, you may be one person, but to one person, you may be the world.

— Bill Wilson

Before his cancer diagnosis, there were at least two parenting tasks that had fallen mostly on David. The first was that he was the one who took the children to the park. I hated parks after Matthew broke his arm falling from a slide. All I could see were hazards in the dangerous slides, monkey bars, and merry-go-rounds. David didn't regard parks in the same way and actually seemed to enjoy them. I had to make myself look away whenever he swung Abby much higher than I ever would.

The second was that David was the designated book reader of the house. He would read the same book over and over to a toddler. Unlike other households where I knew the mother was the main reader, in our house it was to Daddy that the toddlers usually brought their stacks of books. If pressed, I would read, but unless it was a new book we chose together at the library or one of my own personal favorites, I avoided the task. I found repeatedly reading the same story over and over tedious and terribly monotonous. Even I found it odd that I didn't enjoy reading aloud to my toddlers.

Because I have a large family and homeschool, it seemed I should naturally love that sort of thing. I'd spent the better part of a year in 2002 conducting story hour at the local small library where I worked. Everyone commented that it was the ideal job for me, yet I dreaded those sessions and got physically ill from the stress of planning them. I continually sidestepped toddler requests for "one more book" by instead substituting oral made-up stories about wicked little children with names similar to theirs. If my stories didn't suffice, I brought out the coloring books or sent the kids to Daddy. Only when he wasn't available and older siblings were too busy did I reluctantly give in and read aloud.

Each child had a different favorite. One enjoyed every Berenstain Bear book ever written. Another loved the Curious George series. For Abby, it was Clifford the Big Red Dog books. By age three, the first thing Abby said when she woke up each morning was "Where is my daddy?" Inevitably, the next thing out of her mouth was "Read Clifford." And most mornings, David obliged, reading half a dozen Clifford books before getting dressed and leaving for work. One way we'd thought to prepare Abby for her dad's surgery was to warn her that he wouldn't be able to read her books for some time afterward.

We'd done our best to prepare the kids for David's surgery and his subsequent stay in the hospital. We'd never had babysitters before this, but I intended to visit David in the hospital daily, even if it was only for an hour or two. I jumped at the generous offers of babysitting services I got from our oldest daughter Elizabeth, my sisters, and my sister-in-law, Julie. Feasibly, our daughter Rachel could have handled some of the babysitting, but I wasn't sure the youngest two would listen to her if they had to be watched every day. Plus, I felt more confident leaving when I knew an adult would be present. In fact, I felt the most secure on the days when there would be two adults watching and entertaining my children. I knew the kids could be quite a handful, especially the combination of Abby and Katie—both strong-willed children prone to battles over the slightest provocation. The day their uncle Shawn joined my sister Angie in her babysitting duties was especially memorable because Shawn didn't just watch them, he initiated and joined them in sword fights and outdoor play in the yard. Whenever two caretakers were available, one of them inevitably spent a great deal of time in a quiet corner, reading Clifford books to Abby. While Abby reveled in the hours of Clifford stories, she did politely inform my sister Denise that she "did the voices wrong," which Denise knew meant she hadn't read them like David did.

I was pleasantly surprised and slightly chagrined at how easily the children adjusted to having a babysitter every day. Abby quickly discovered which babysitter would read her countless Clifford books. When my sister Angie tried to slip in other books to keep her own son Andrew entertained, Abby repeatedly thrust her chosen books at her and stated, "No, read Clifford." Angie knew why, and so did I. My soft-hearted sisters naturally gave in to Abby's demands because it was those books that reminded Abby of her daddy.

The second day Dan and I visited the hospital together, we found David in much the same state as the night before. Neither one of us could stand to see him in such pain, so our visit was very brief, even though we both felt guilty leaving him alone. I felt torn between wanting to be there with him and hating to see him like that. When we left the room after a few minutes, the nurse at the ICU desk could see how difficult it had been for us. A tiny thing with a sweet face, she gave me a hug as I started crying outside of his room.

"How can I leave him? Will he feel like I'm abandoning him?" I asked her.

"He needs his rest. He'll be sleeping a lot," she reassured me. "Sometimes it is harder for the patient to have visitors because they try so hard to respond and struggle to stay awake."

Whether that was true or not, her words made it easier to leave. As Dan and I turned to go, she added, "Call us anytime you want. Give us a call when you want to see how he is doing or to have us tell him that you love him."

I gave her the letter I had written, asking to have it attached to the front of his chart. I had no doubts about her wonderful care of my husband, but I liked knowing that she and all the other nurses could learn something about David when he was unable to talk.

After that, I visited the hospital by myself, staggering my visits with Dan's so that David wouldn't be alone as long. Each day he showed some improvement.

On David's fifth day in ICU, Elizabeth had her first chance to visit him. Dan and my son-in-law, Ben, had agreed to be the designated babysitters for the afternoon, watching all of the kids together at my house. Elizabeth's daughter, my granddaughter Rebecca, was three months younger than our Abby, and little Jacob had just turned one and still nursed often. She'd never left both of them alone with Ben for more than an hour, so she was understandably nervous, but her need to visit her father overrode her concerns. When we arrived at the hospital, the nurses were just getting ready to move David to surgical services on another floor. David's eyes brightened when he saw his oldest daughter. He pointed at the nurse who was leaving the room and gave a "thumbs down." Elizabeth and I both laughed out loud. I knew David wouldn't want Elizabeth viewing his struggle to get on his feet or his shuffling gait as he walked partway to the other room, so I took her to a lounge while the staff settled him in. It was then she commented on the distinct smell I'd also noticed on the ward: a sickly sweet odor that might politely be described as flatulence mixed with honey. I didn't realize then that it was from the cans of the liquid nutrition that I would soon come to know so well. Once they started David on his tube feedings, that smell would remain in my nostrils even when I escaped the hospital. I would wake up in the middle of the night and wonder where the pungent odor was coming from, only to realize it was from inside my own nose.

I thought the younger children were handling David's absence amazingly well. The various babysitters reported few problems, and my children seemed to thrive on the individual attention they received. I was inevitably punished for my repeated absences though, by their negative and clingy behavior after the babysitters left. I came home exhausted from my hospital visits but felt the need to be wholly there for the children, despite their constant demands.

I'd started writing in a journal for David the second day after his surgery. I missed him so much, especially in the middle of the night. Since I couldn't talk to him, I'd write to him. One morning I wrote:

> *The kids are doing okay. The diversion of having others come to take care of them helps, but when I come home, all hell breaks loose. I know. Deal with it, right? They are so used to having me here all day, every day, and then they vie for my attention when I do come home. Especially Katie and Abby. And they really don't understand what is going on—that Daddy is fighting for his life, and Mommy needs to be there to help him. And, frankly, I'm kind of a wreck right now. They see me crying and it confuses them.*

Nights, especially, were difficult for me. I had household chores to catch up on and children to get ready for bed. Several times I came home to find that someone else had done laundry or dishes, which helped tremendously, but there was always supper to be made and toys to be picked up. This was also the time when friends or family members phoned me for updates on David's condition. If I didn't get a phone call from David's brother Keith, I called him. During the time that David couldn't speak, it helped me to hear Keith's similar voice and mannerisms of speech. Besides, Keith was the one person I could talk to without crying. He wasn't much for putting feelings into words and said so during one of our conversations. The night I called distraught over David's apparent pain, Keith's voice cracked when he told me to tell David that he cared about him. I knew what he wasn't saying: that he loved his brother.

I wasn't getting much sleep. I would fall asleep with the three youngest little girls in our bedroom and wake up throughout the night, wondering how David was doing and if he felt abandoned. The nurses at the ICU had gotten used to me phoning each night to have them tell David I loved him and each morning to let him know when I would be able to visit that day. When David moved to the surgical services floor, the nurses looked at me strangely when I asked if I could do the same thing there. Because of that, I felt uncomfortable calling more than once a day. Wondering if my letter had followed him to the new floor, I asked one of the student nurses if it was still in his chart. Her eyes lit up when she said yes. She commented that she wished everyone would do the same for patients who couldn't talk.

On the sixth morning of David's hospitalization, Abby woke up asking, "Where is my daddy?"

My heart heavy, I answered, "In the hospital."

Then she repeated the question louder, this time pausing dramatically between each word, "Where. Is. My. Daddy."

"In the hospital," I said again. "Remember? He had an operation, but he will get better soon."

She leaned in close, put her small hands on either side of my face, looked straight into my eyes and whispered, "No. Where is my daddy?"

It dawned on me then that with her three-year-old level of understanding, she might be thinking she would never see her daddy again. Because he had been gone for so many days and she wasn't allowed to see him, in her mind, he might not even exist anymore. Her beautiful brown eyes that reminded me so much of her father's never left my face as she looked for reassurance. I hugged her tightly and whispered back, "He's in the hospital. Really he is. And I promise that he will get better and come home soon."

Later that day, when Elizabeth took her turn babysitting her younger sister, she was swinging her outside when Abby piped up, "I have a daddy."

"Yes, you do," Elizabeth answered. "He's my daddy, too. He'll be coming home soon."

By this time, David had gotten proficient at conversing by writing on a dry erase board. While still very weak, he was in less pain. I noticed him pushing his morphine button less often. Still, our visits mostly consisted of me sitting on a chair near the bed holding his hand as he drifted in and out of sleep.

The majority of the nurses were wonderful, but the one at the front desk always seemed irritated whenever David rang the call bell on her watch. During one of my first visits to the surgical services floor, David had to go to the bathroom. The only person available was this woman, so we hesitated. Finally, unable to wait any longer, he pushed the call button, but after a few more minutes, I realized I was going to have to help get him to his feet to use the dispos-able urinal. Positioning him upright was a job in itself with all the wires hooked up to him. When he finished and the nurse still hadn't appeared, I rubbed lotion on his back in the same way I'd seen the nurses do and then helped him get into the bed. When she finally did respond, the nurse didn't even apologize for her delay. Over the next several days, we got quite proficient at this maneuver, making me wonder if the delays were deliberate—to force me to learn to care for David's needs. I worried that, in my absence, David's calls wouldn't elicit an immediate response, but he nodded when I asked him if the nurses usually came quicker when I wasn't there.

I felt very tender toward David, unaccustomed to seeing him so vulnerable. It was as though I was able to see, for the first time in a long time, the best of David: his strength in dealing with pain and the annoying tracheotomy tube, his gentleness as he held my hand, his concerned questions about the kids written on the board. Without his ability to speak, our stilted conversations left me with a heightened sense of having to learn about my husband in other ways. I scrutinized his movements and eyes for clues to what he needed, guessing his feet were cold if he pointed at them, or that his blankets were too heavy on the wound on his abdomen where the feeding tube protruded. It gave me a real sense of satisfaction when he nodded and relaxed after I adjusted his pillows or made him comfortable in some way. I envied the nurses the opportunities they had to rub lotion on his back or help him to a chair when I was not there. I relished the times I could be there to do those things.

I surprised both of us one day when, looking at him, I blurted out, "You're beautiful." He shook his head no, like I was crazy.

Then I stood up and leaned over, hugging him the best I could with all the tubes and wires. Blushing, I whispered, "You are beautiful. I want to make love to you."

He smiled, but rolled his eyes, like I was being silly.

Finally, I understood how David had felt after my emergency c-section. I was in the hospital bed with an IV and catheter, still reeling from the shock to my system, when he'd blurted out, "I want to make love to you." At the time, I'd reared back and brushed him away, not understanding how he could say such a thing when I felt so debilitated and weak. Now I knew exactly what he had meant. He loved me and wanted everything to be normal.

I wrote in our journal that night:

> I told you in the hospital today that I want to make love to you and you looked at me a bit strangely. Remember saying the exact same thing to me shortly after my emergency c-section? I just thought you were a "nut" then. Now I feel the same way.
>
> It's because I want everything to be normal, and it's the closest I can get to you. I want to crawl up in your hospital bed with you, wrap my arms around you, and crawl under your skin. It might sound crazy to the person in the hospital gown, but it makes perfect sense to me now.

My visits with David became a ritual of sorts. Each morning, dressing for the hospital visit, I took a shower, smoothing fragrant lotion on my arms and legs afterward. I spent an inordinate amount of time on my makeup and hair and in choosing my clothes. I'd stand before the closet, searching for something, anything, that didn't resemble the standard mom-at-home uniform of leggings or jeans and a loose shirt that I had been wearing for so many years. My choices were pretty limited. I didn't spend much on my wardrobe and had relied on the sales at a local thrift shop and my sister's consignment store's annual bag sales for the majority of my clothing. Now, suddenly, I wanted to look as lovely to David as he looked to me. Each day when I visited, I gazed into his brown eyes and saw the man I had fallen in love with. Without the trappings of our busy household and the distraction of children, I spent time in that hospital room getting to know my husband and falling in love with him all over again.

I was courting my own husband.

Chapter Five

The Next Step

Courage is being afraid but going on anyhow.
—Dan Rather

Dr. Gordon was "real people." David and I both instinctively knew it upon our first meeting. Years before, David and I had coined the phrase "real people" to refer to those we considered the salt of the earth. It was the highest honor an acquaintance could receive: to become real people in our eyes, as opposed to someone pretentious. We'd counted my father as real people, along with my brother John and our son Dan. While their type didn't usually whine or complain, they could have the unnerving habit of blunt honesty. They were the best people to go to for advice, as long as you were ready to hear the truth.

Besides coming up with a phrase to label our favorite kinds of people, our family also had the odd habit of privately nicknaming some of those people we crossed paths with in our daily life. There was "The Frogman" with the deep voice from Dan's old paper route, the postal worker we named "Steven" because he looked like a Steven (even though his real name was Randy), the UPS driver we dubbed "Larry," and a cashier with tight curls and an equally tight expression we named "Curly Head." Only once had a child accidentally used a nickname in public, calling a grocery store worker "Fake Lyle" within his hearing. The worker looked and acted so much like their Uncle Lyle that they had dubbed him "Fake Lyle." I blushed furiously when the man asked why my daughter had called him Fake Lyle, but it turned out my explanation amused him, and the next time my brother (the real Lyle), a Wonder Bread truck driver, delivered bread to his store, Fake Lyle shared the story with him. Before long, they were bantering back and forth, joking about which of them was the "fake" one.

The day before David was to come home, we were to meet with both a radiation oncologist and a medical oncologist in his hospital room to discuss future treatment of his cancer. When Dr. Gordon strode into the room, her bright, discerning eyes first acknowledged David, then me, before she pulled up a chair and sat in front of us. After introducing herself as the radiation oncologist from the nearby cancer center, she asked us a few questions about ourselves and our lifestyle, seeming genuinely interested and putting us at ease. My mind raced as I answered her questions. David still had trouble speaking, even though his breathing tube had been removed on the eighth day of his stay in the hospital. His voice was hoarse and his throat tired easily, so he let me do most of the talking.

Dr. Gordon pulled out charts from the file folder she held. Finally, the moment of truth had come. I'd been anticipating the news of the biopsy of the lymph nodes and a more definitive idea of the stage of David's cancer. I hadn't even told David there was a possibility the cancer had not been contained by the lymph nodes. Dr. Gordon showed us the chart as she explained exactly how David's cancer had been staged. Of the thirty-two lymph nodes removed, two contained cancer cells. The one large lymph node that had concerned Dr. Alt measured at four centimeters and did indeed show extracapsular extension, or ECE, which meant that cancer cells were left behind in the tissue. This put David's cancer at stage IV—the most serious and advanced stage. As Dr. Gordon explained, there was no way to know if those escaped cancer cells had been eradicated by Dr. Alt's surgery or how far or where they had traveled. That meant that David's best chance of ridding his body of cancer was to undergo both radiation and chemotherapy. She paused to see if we had any questions. We were too stunned by the news to reply. We had expected radiation, but a chemotherapy regimen wasn't a part of the original plans. We couldn't help but remember how Dr. Alt had described chemotherapy during our initial visit with him, not to mention the dire comment he'd made about people dying from the chemo itself.

"There is good news," she said as she handed a sheaf of papers to me. "David qualifies for a clinical trial which gives him his best chance at surviving this type of cancer." She explained the Phase II trial and what it entailed, then warned that this regimen would be hard on David.

"You will hate me by the end of the treatment," she warned.

She asked that we carefully look over the papers and make a decision about participating in the trial, promising that either way David would get "the standard of care" at their center, which basically meant the treatment would be the same no matter where he went. Before shaking our hands and leaving the room, she reiterated that we should think long and hard before making a decision.

As much as I wanted to run after her and immediately sign David up for anything that would give him even a slight benefit in beating this cancer, I knew we needed to do our own research and, ultimately, it had to be David's decision. Dr. Gordon had assured us we had time to explore our options as it would be at least four weeks before treatment could begin. It spoke volumes about her that four weeks later, when she ran into David and me for the first time since our visit in the hospital, she greeted David by name and remembered that we had eight children and homeschooled.

After Dr. Gordon's friendly and informative meeting, our subsequent visit with the medical oncologist that same morning left us disappointed and confused. Dr. Holm explained very little about why David needed chemotherapy and seemed to assume that David would be participating in the clinical trial. Her flamboyant style left a positive impression on us, but her bedside manner seemed distant, despite a deliberate attempt to portray herself as a caring doctor by sitting on the bed next to David and occasionally putting a hand on his leg in a show of empathy. Privately, we would call her "The Queen" for the remainder of his treatment because of her regal stature and beautiful clothing. We amused ourselves with predictions of what her next outfit would be and found ourselves sorely disappointed once when she wore a simple black pantsuit. Our secret nickname for her remained until post-cancer checkups when her demeanor abruptly warmed.

If we hadn't dealt with Dr. Gordon initially, we might have started looking for a second opinion. As it was, our gut feeling was to trust Dr. Gordon and follow her recommendations. If that meant dealing with a medical oncologist that we didn't initially feel comfortable with, then that was a small price to pay for the opportunity to have Dr. Gordon as our doctor. By the end of David's treatment, we would find ourselves admiring "The Queen" as well.

We hadn't blindly followed medical advice for several years. We weren't about to now, despite my urge to do whatever Dr. Gordon suggested. Dealing with my chronic illness that had been difficult to diagnose had changed us profoundly. The disillusionment with the medical establishment was fueled by a legion of doctors who'd begun viewing me with a wariness bordering on disbelief when I'd searched to find out what was wrong with me back in 1992.

We'd crossed paths with other doctors with less-than-stellar bedside manners in the interim since my chronic illness. Initially, we lived too far away from Dr. Tomas, who had diagnosed my CFS, to use him as our family doctor. For several years, our children saw other doctors for their checkups and illnesses. One weekend, I called one of those doctors for my own care as I was suffering with a raging breast infection. I'd had several infections while nursing baby Matthew and knew the signs and symptoms. Trying to avoid an emergency room charge, I talked to the doctor on-call and explained that I had yet another breast infection—my fourth in five months. When he asked how old the baby was, I said, "Six months."

He retorted nastily, "No wonder you keep getting breast infections. He's too old to be nursed!"

This was the same doctor who'd dismissed me airily in the emergency room a year before that when I'd had a panic attack during the worst of my undiagnosed illness.

"Give her a shot," he'd told the nurse gruffly, then pulled my husband aside and told him to stop coddling me because there was nothing wrong with me.

I hated having to deal with these kinds of doctors, and as soon as we moved closer to Dr. Tomas, we started seeing him exclusively. He was a keenly intelligent doctor who seemed to admire that same trait in his own patients. He always took the time to thoroughly listen and knew I conducted extensive research before making major medical decisions. Unlike doctors we'd dealt with before, he supported our right as parents to make decisions regarding our children's health care. Since my chronic illness, I'd made the unorthodox decision to delay our infants' vaccination schedules and forgo some immunizations altogether. While he didn't agree with my concerns about the long-term effects of immunizations, he respected my right to make an informed decision.

Only two years prior to David's cancer diagnosis, we'd had to make another difficult decision regarding a series of rabies shots when David woke up to find a bat crawling on him. By the time we'd found the dead bat's body, its brain was too decomposed to test, so we had to consider the very real possibility that the bat had rabies and had bitten him while he was asleep. I'd called the Iowa Department of Health and was told that bat bites are so small you cannot see them, and if asleep, you might not feel the bite. Because rabies is always fatal, we were informed that David definitely needed rabies shots. We got conflicting views on whether or not Abby and I, the other two people in the room, should have the series of shots. Because one was a sleeping infant, standard recommendation was for the series of shots for her, too. The three of us ended up having the six-week series of shots. It made for an interesting situation when all of us simultaneously experienced the unusual side effect of waking up at two in the morning and being unable to fall back asleep.

Now we were faced with a serious decision regarding David's continued treatment plan. Naturally, because of our previous medical experience, we weren't likely to just jump at a clinical drug trial for David until we felt sure it was the best route to take.

I started researching alternative, complementary, and standard treatments for cancer the evening of our meeting with Dr. Gordon. I spent several hours online over the next few days, reading about the expected side effects of radiation and chemotherapy and searching for information on alternative treatments.

While doing this research, I found several references to the plight of a sixteen-year-old homeschooled young man, Abraham Cherrix. He lived in Virginia and had already completed chemotherapy treatment for Hodgkin's Disease and was now facing a second round of chemotherapy since the disease had returned. Cherrix and his parents were fighting the courts for the right to refuse chemotherapy and to try alternative treatments. They'd started a regimen of herbal remedies and an organic diet. The court system was originally poised to remove the young man from his family's home on the grounds of medical neglect. The judge eventually ruled that the boy and his parents had done their research and allowed them to continue their desired treatment, along with low-dose radiation treatments under the care of an oncologist open to alternative treatments. I found this intriguing and delved into some of the websites that discussed herbal and natural treatments.

Around this time, too, the litany of advice from others began. I tried to remain open to anything even remotely hopeful in regards to alternative or complementary treatments for cancer. After all, we had hardly been traditional in our approaches to medical treatments the past few years. I'd begun using cabbage leaf compresses with great success to alleviate plugged milk ducts when I was nursing, lecithin and liver cleansing tablets for my gallbladder woes, and Echinacea to ward off illness after we'd been exposed to a cold.

But when it came to cancer, I had a difficult time considering alternative treatments in place of radiation and chemotherapy. I found there were plenty of websites and books devoted to bashing mainstream cancer treatments and promoting alternative methods ranging from special diets to herbal concoctions that promised to cure the disease. We already agreed with the doctors that chemotherapy and radiation were crucial in beating the cancer. After all, there were ten million Americans still alive because of standard cancer treatments. Frankly, I wanted to find information that would convince me David didn't need either radiation or chemotherapy. I wanted to discover something that wouldn't be so hard on his body but would still fight the cancer. Unfortunately, I didn't find it. I saw a huge difference in websites with pages of testimonials versus those with scientific statistics that proved the successful results of traditional cancer treatments. What I began looking for then was something that would alleviate side effects and perhaps help prevent further cancer cell growth.

I pored over books and articles on cancer treatments and friends and relatives sent plenty more our way. Even complete strangers approached us with advice when they found out David had cancer. We would hear about oils, juices, and herb concoctions that promised to kill cancer cells. Later, I would research some of these to decide if they were worth using as dietary supplements, but none of the claims left me feeling confident enough to use them in conjunction with, or as a substitute to, traditional treatment. After much discussion and research, we decided it was very important not to use anything that might alter the effects of the standard treatments.

I also wasn't completely confident about the decision to go with a Phase II trial for David. A couple of the books I'd read warned against signing up for clinical trials at all, suggesting that patients who did so were nothing more than guinea pigs. I didn't see it that way. Oral cancer had a high recidivism rate. The drug agent cetuximab(C225), commonly referred to as Erbitux, had been used for years for colon cancer, but the FDA had recently approved it for use on oral cancer patients. Erbitux seemed to be promising in helping to prevent future tumor growth. The trial that Dr. Gordon had told us about was to study which chemotherapy drug it was most effective with, docetaxel or cisplatin. From my research, I'd concluded that Erbitux could have a significant impact on preventing a reoccurrence. It had made a difference in the reoccurrence rate of colon cancer. It could prove to make a difference in the survival rate of oral cancer, too. I wanted David to have that extra chance.

I didn't want to be the one to make this decision, but David was in no shape to make it alone. Since I did the research on the computer, I read pertinent information aloud to him from the websites.

After all this research, I was convinced that Dr. Gordon was correct. The clinical drug trial was David's best chance. He agreed.

I was convinced of something else, too. David would be hit hard by chemotherapy and radiation. Adding Erbitux to the mix would do more than just give him a better chance at survival—it would exacerbate the side effects of both treatments and add a few additional side effects to the mix. David had a rough road ahead of him.

Chapter Six

Bringing Daddy Home

Any fool can be a Father, but it takes a real man to be a Daddy!

—**Philip Whitmore Sr.**

One of the worst things a husband can say when he sees his wife vacuuming or dusting is "Who's coming?" insinuating that the only time she cleans is when she expects company.

I was annoyed by this question when David or the kids saw me vacuuming behind the furniture or dusting the end tables. What was even more irritating was that nine times out of ten they were correct, and my frenzied housecleaning was in response to an expected visitor.

You might say that during my years raising small children, I was a less-than-stellar housekeeper. I did the bare minimum to keep my house clean, letting things like sock matching or dusting build up until the unmatched socks or dust bunnies threatened to take over the house. I liked to tell myself that the children and I were too busy to bother with little things like the general upkeep of the house. In fact, at times I caught myself taking a perverse sort of pleasure and pride at how we were "too creative" to be tidy.

To my credit, there were aspects of running an active household I was very adept at, such as keeping our books and school supplies well organized, filling our bathroom shelves with freshly washed and line-dried towels, and stockpiling health and beauty items I'd gotten for free or nearly free with coupons. As a homeschooling family, however, we really were busy with our respective interests and activities that involve a lot of messy art materials, reams of paper, and stacks of books and magazines. Pairing socks and dusting were usually at the bottom of our to-do lists, and an energetic toddler meant there were always toys strewn about.

Before David's surgery, I'd found myself frantically cleaning closets and catching up on all the little household chores I never seemed to get around to. The frenetic activity reminded me of what I had always thought of as the nesting instinct the weeks prior to each of my baby's births. This time, however, it seemed more like nervous energy to keep my mind off cancer.

Somehow I'd managed to keep my house clean and organized the entire length of David's hospital stay. The legion of babysitters helped on that front, straightening up the living room and kitchen after their respective stints with childcare. Rachel pitched in more than usual, too. Still, the lion's share of housekeeping fell on my shoulders. I'd wake up early each morning, long before the children, just to have some alone time to check my e-mails or work at my desk. Then I'd head into the kitchen and make tea and toast before picking up stray dishes and toys around the house. Once the children were up, I'd quickly run the vacuum cleaner over the rugs. Then I'd get Abby dressed and fed before heading upstairs to perform my own transformation before the mirror.

When each day's babysitter arrived, even the playroom was neat and clean, ready for a day of unfettered fun with aunts or cousins. By the time I returned home late each afternoon, I was exhausted but determined to spend some quality time with my children, who never seemed to miss me until I returned. I was also determined to keep up with the house, which usually meant straightening up again before the kids and I went to bed.

I knew how tough it was to come home after a hospital stay, even though my postpartum stays had been brief. I'd felt emotionally and physically fragile after surgery and knew the difficulty David would face, coming from a quiet hospital to a house full of rambunctious children. My main concern was to make the transition as easy as possible for him, and I was certain that arriving home to a clean house would lessen the impact on his emotional state.

On the morning of July 22, I took extra pains dressing nicely and cleaning the living room. It was very hot and humid, so I ran the air conditioner while I worked. For the last time that month, I would be heading to the hospital alone. David was being released and would finally be coming home. My hands actually shook as I got dressed that morning, with anticipation, nerves, or both, I wasn't sure. I even suggested to the children that they play outside for most of the morning, just so the house would stay as neat as I'd left it.

I had a short detour on the way, stopping at the Humane Society to drop off several kittens we'd discovered in the ditch that week. Somehow, on the way to Dubuque to pick David up, they escaped from the box I'd brought them in. By the time I struggled to capture them all and return them to the container, I was sweaty and disheveled. On the drive to the hospital, I occasionally smelled cat feces. I hoped the smell wouldn't be noticed by either David or the nurse who wheeled him out. I arrived at the hospital and quickly brushed my hair in the elevator, checking my makeup in the compact I had in my purse.

When I got to his room, I found David alone, sitting in a chair, dressed in the clothing he'd worn when he arrived, his hair freshly washed for the first time since the surgery. He looked handsome to me despite the vivid and oozing scar on his neck. I stood expectantly at his side, and after greeting me effusively, he looked down at my feet.

"What's that on your foot?" he asked.

I looked down. There, on the top of my blue sandal was a huge brown splat of cat poop. Evidently, one of the kittens had defecated on my shoe, and in my rush to get to the hospital, I hadn't even noticed. Stifling a nervous giggle, I hurried into the bathroom to clean up before anyone else could see it. I couldn't imagine the nurses releasing their charge to a woman doused in cat poop.

It wasn't long before nurses were bustling back and forth in the room, readying their patient for dismissal and gathering supplies for our trip home, including a tall metal pole to hang feeding bags from and bins of dressings for his wounds. As I looked at all the supplies, my throat went dry and my stomach clenched. Would the nurses rethink David's discharge if they knew they were sending their well-cared-for patient to a hotbed of activity and noise? I was unsure of my ability to properly care for David. Would I be able to change the dressing on his feeding tube and neck area? Do the feedings without the help of a nurse? Unlike my discharges from the hospital, this one seemed to be happening too quickly. Paperwork was being thrust in my hands by the accommodating nurses. When I glanced at the sheet of drug orders and saw the sheer number of different drugs David was taking, I wondered what would happen if I forgot one of his medicines or inadvertently overdosed him.

Then, as I looked up from the sheaf of papers, my eyes met David's, and just as suddenly as the anxiety had risen, it disappeared completely. His brown eyes that had been clouded by pain and medication in the past days were now bright. The smile on his face was huge. I smiled back. David was coming home. We waited in heady anticipation while a nurse went to get a wheelchair.

"You're going to start your new life today," the nurse trilled as she came back in the room with the wheelchair.

"You're like a caterpillar in a cocoon ready to become a butterfly," she continued as she assisted him into the chair.

I led the way out of the room, pushing the cart full of nutritional formula boxes ahead of me and pulling the metal stand behind me. I could hear the nurse's musical refrain continue as we headed to the elevators.

"You are both like butterflies, flying off to your new life."

The litany of cocoon, butterfly, and new life continued in the elevator. By the time we got off the elevator I felt like running to get the van. I reluctantly left David in the care of the singing nurse and rushed to the parking lot. As I drove up to the visitor's entrance, I could see the nurse's lips moving, and I wondered if she was still repeating the same phrase, over and over, to David. He wasn't really listening. He had eyes only for me as I drove the van up to the entrance. I jumped out and quickly loaded up the boxes of nutritional formula, bins of medical dressings, and supplies. After giving her a quick goodbye hug, David let the nurse help him into the van, giving me a knowing smile apparently sharing my amusement at her butterfly spiel.

My heart surged with joy as I got back into the driver's side. I wanted to take David home.

I wanted to get away from that nurse.

As we left the hospital parking lot, we heard it at the same time: a soft mewing sound coming from underneath the seat. I'd missed one of the kittens! We were giddy with laughter by the time we stopped at the Humane Society again.

Before we left town, David mentioned that he didn't have clothes to wear when he got home. I'd already thought of that since he'd need the forgiving elastic on his sore abdomen, and he was already wearing the only pair of elastic waist shorts he owned. I'd brought a ten-dollar rebate check from the Shopko store and planned on looking for shorts there. I was going to run in by myself, but David didn't seem to want to be away from me for even that short time. We went in together and I pushed David around the store in a wheel-chair. I headed to the athletic clothing section and pointed out a pair of gray, elastic waist shorts with the logo of his favorite team (the Iowa Hawkeyes) on it. They were on sale for $11.97. David nodded that he liked them, but protested when I reached for a matching t-shirt at the same price.

"No, that's too much," he said.

I suddenly felt very sad. David thought $24 was too much to spend on himself? Like mine, David's wardrobe had pretty much consisted of thrift store finds since we'd had children. I hadn't minded for myself, but now I minded for David. He worked hard supporting his family. He used to buy himself new clothing before we'd gotten married. We'd been able to find him nice quality brand-name clothing secondhand, and he always looked nice. Still, I couldn't shake that sense of sadness. Was he just being thrifty, or had he gotten to the point where he didn't feel like he deserved new things?

For the most part, no one would guess our income status just by looking at us. Because of ready access to garage sales, thrift stores, and consignment stores, our children were usually dressed well. When I was a child growing up in poverty, my limited ward-robe of two faded dresses with let-down hems, thick acrylic socks, and brown boy's shoes served to categorize me as "the poor girl" in a Catholic grade school full of little girls in puffed sleeved dresses, crisp white bobby-socks, and shiny, black Mary Janes. In contrast, my children had drawers spilling over with quality name-brand clothing. And while my own wardrobe was limited, I had stocked up on expensive nursing tops the past few years for ease and comfort in public breastfeeding. No one seeing me and my brood in public would immediately peg us as low-income simply because of our clothing.

Even visiting our home, a person would not automatically assume our lower-income status. The 100-year-old brick home we rented looked cozy and comfortable, and the faded rugs matched our secondhand furniture nicely. Through years of hunting down deals, I'd managed to decorate an apple kitchen and a rose-themed bathroom on a garage sale budget.

Vehicles, however, were another matter. We'd always driven older, used vehicles that we paid cash for, and most of them accurately reflected our financial status. One of David's cars we'd affectionately dubbed "Rust Bucket" because there was more rust showing than white paint. It turned out to be one of the most reliable cars we'd ever owned, so it was easy to ignore the rust. We'd driven another car that necessitated carrying a hammer to occasionally hit the starter if it had landed on a certain spot when we turned the engine off. Until we could afford repairs, I'd felt a real sense of resourcefulness being able to get it started by myself with the hammer when needed. As long as our vehicles ran and got us where we needed to go, what they looked like mattered very little to me. Repairing vehicles was something else. If we didn't have the money or David wasn't able to fix it himself, things could get pretty tense around the homestead, which is why reliability mattered so much more than appearance with our vehicles. Most of the time our vehicle foibles only served to amuse me, but what if David had stopped being amused and started feeling ashamed of not having money?

Buying used clothing and furniture and driving older vehicles seemed a small price for us to pay for the opportunity for me to be able to stay home with our children. I knew our choices to allow God to plan our family and the subsequent result of having a large family was misunderstood by many people. But our religious convictions meant we also believed that God would provide for our needs. And he always had, though his provisions might not be up to par with what many in our materialistic society deemed necessary or even adequate.

Though little about our lower-income lifestyle bothered me, I did know what it meant to feel ashamed, mostly from my child-hood experiences in school. Luckily, in twenty-seven years, I could remember only one time when I'd actually felt ashamed about driving an old vehicle. A couple of years before, on a beastly hot summer day, I'd loaded the four youngest children into our 1988 Dodge Caravan for a trip to the grocery store. We drove with the windows down since the air conditioner had long since ceased working. Upon our arrival to the store, I unloaded the kids and slammed the side door shut, only to have the running board come loose on one side and crash to the ground. I tried to pull the other side off but it was secured with two large bolts, and no matter how much I pulled or twisted, it wouldn't come loose.

The kids and I stood there for a moment, staring at the vehicle. It seemed a ridiculous situation.

"How are we going to get home?" one of them asked. "We can't drive with that thing dragging on the ground."

"Never mind," I told them as they stood there in the hot sun waiting for me to fix everything. I determinedly strapped baby Abby into the backpack.

"We'll ask the guys in the store if they have some kind of tool I can use to loosen this."

I went through the store quickly, stopping to ask each of the male employees if they had a tool in their car that I could remove my running board with. Every single one shook his head no.

By the time the children and I finished shopping, I'd come up with an idea. We loaded our groceries into the van and walked over to the Pamida store only a parking lot away. I bought a huge roll of duct tape and we returned to the van. The children watched intently as I kneeled down on the hot cement of the parking lot and carefully duct-taped the entire running board to the side of the van, using generous amounts of the sticky stuff. We all laughed at how funny the van looked with the running board taped to it. The end product looked like something from one of their dad's favorite television programs, *The Red Green Show*, where the leader of the Possum Lodge rigs up crazy inventions with his roll of duct tape.

Still smiling, I turned to the sound of a car pulling up next to us. As I rose from the ground, the baby still strapped to me in my backpack, I wanted to share the absurdity of our situation with someone else.

An impeccably dressed woman stepped out of the clean and shiny new car next to us. She stood there looking down at the duct tape on my van, then her eyes rested on me with my by-now rumpled skirt and sweaty face. I smiled at her as her eyes moved to the three children standing next to me.

"Think it will hold until I get home?" I laughed as I gestured towards the van with the roll of duct tape still in my hand. She didn't respond. Her eyes were cold as she continued to stare at us in such a way that my smile soon disappeared and I flushed with embarrassment. She stood there several moments longer, just staring, a clear look of distaste on her face.

Flustered, I turned away from her and quickly herded the children through the passenger door of the van. Even facing away from her, I could sense her glaring at my back. When I turned to sit down on the sidewalk to get the backpack off, she'd finally disappeared into the store but had left a palpable air of disgust behind her. I wanted to laugh again at the silliness of the whole situation but instead felt like crying. I was also angry for letting someone else make me feel ashamed when I really had nothing to feel ashamed of. I resisted the strong urge to duct-tape her car door shut, and I left.

I wondered if other people sometimes made David feel like that. If they had, he'd never mentioned it. I wanted David to have new things and to feel like he deserved them, because he did. A pair of shorts and a cotton t-shirt was not going to make or break our budget.

"We're buying them," I stated firmly as I put them in the small cart in the front of the wheelchair. "You need something comfortable, and you deserve them. Besides, the rebate check will pay for half of this outfit."

Once again that day, David's smile was huge and genuine, and I saw him finger the cotton material with pleasure as we headed to the checkout.

Our four youngest children were outside in the yard as we pulled into the driveway. Matthew and Emily ran to the van, but Katie and Abby held back until I got out of the driver's side, and then they ran to me, hiding their faces in my skirt, barely looking at their dad. They were uncharacteristically quiet. David greeted the children effusively in a hoarse voice they didn't recognize. I'd warned them he would sound funny, but from their expressions I knew they weren't prepared for this strange voice coming from their beloved daddy. As he reached out to pat their heads, Katie and Abby shyly ducked away, still sneaking glances at him. They clung to my side as they warily watched his labored walk to the porch.

As we entered the house, I was pleased to see it had remained as clean as I'd left it. David sunk gratefully into the chair we had set up for him in the corner of the room in front of the hallway door. The children still hung back, unsure. As David relaxed, Matthew and Emily brought in the medical supplies and boxes and then stood expectantly in front of him. I pushed the end table closer to his chair, busying myself setting up the things he'd had near his bed in the hospital: a paper cup of ice water, small sponges on sticks designed to freshen and wet his mouth, and fresh water in a container for his tube feedings. Then I taped the drug list on the door behind his chair, where it would stay for several weeks during his recovery from surgery. As I did these things, I talked out loud to the kids, explaining the purpose of all the paraphernalia. Abby and Katie seemed particularly interested in the green sponge sticks, and their eyes reflected their wonder and awe as their daddy dipped one in water and demonstrated their use, wetting the inside of his mouth.

I saw Abby tentatively smile and reach out to touch David's leg. He looked different, he sounded different, but her daddy was finally home.

Chapter Seven

Not Tonight, Honey, I've Got Cancer

According to the Bible, the marriage act
is more than a physical act. It is an act
of sharing. It is an act of communion. It
is an act of total self-giving wherein the
husband gives himself completely to the
wife, and the wife gives herself to the
husband in such a way that the two actually become one flesh.

—Wayne Mack

It was wonderful to sleep next to David again. On his first night home, he replaced Katie in our king-size bed. The little girls made up beds on our floor since ours was the only upstairs room with an air conditioner, and we were still enduring a heat wave with temperatures that didn't get below 85 degrees, even at night. Matthew and Rachel remained in their own stifling hot rooms, despite my invitation to join us in the "welcome home" slumber party in our bedroom.

That first night, I fell asleep holding David's hand but slept fitfully, waking up frequently and listening for a moan or any sign of discomfort coming from him. Only once during that first night did I have to get up to give him a painkiller in his feeding tube, otherwise he slept soundly.

It didn't take long to get into a routine of sorts in caring for David's needs. The day after he was discharged, a home health aide came to our home and showed me how to change the dressings around his feeding tube and neck. After two more home health aide visits, I was confidently setting up tube feedings, changing dressings, and administering his many medications, efficiently checking off the daily doses on the chart I'd made.

At first, I drove David to Dubuque to see the surgeon every few days for checkups. The neck wound needed to heal from the inside out, so Dr. Alt packed gauze into the wound so it would stay open while it healed. After he removed the dressing during one appointment, he showed me how I needed to clean the area.

"Can you do this a few times a day?" he asked as he demonstrated. He inserted the cotton-covered end of an abnormally long stick deep into David's neck wound and began twisting it.

I felt a little lightheaded as I watched. Did I have a choice? Could I call a home health aide to come to our house a couple of times a day to clean the wound? Could we drive to Dubuque every day and have the doctor clean it?

Dr. Alt looked at me expectantly, waiting for an answer.

"Yes, I can do that," I said with more bravado that I actually felt.

The first time was the hardest. Inserting the stick inside my husband's neck slowly, I watched his eyes for any pain I might be inflicting on him. I shouldn't have worried. The area of healing was numb and David said he barely felt it. After a few days, it became just another routine part of the care I was giving my spouse.

Caring for David's physical needs kept me busy, and reminded me of the early weeks of caring for a newborn, not just because of the feedings every three hours but because of the fatigue-induced fog that blurred the days together.

Besides caring for David, I still had the younger children to care for as well. Some days I felt like the proverbial chicken with its head cut off. My parents used to butcher chickens, so I knew all about headless chickens. As a child, I had to help corner and catch the squawking chickens for my dad, who would cut off their heads with a quick action of the ax on an old stump of a tree. Some of the chickens flopped around on the ground for a while afterwards. When their movements ceased, my dad dipped them into scalding hot water to loosen their feathers. Occasionally, however, one of the headless chickens would get back on its feet and start to run around aimlessly. I never forgot the sight, and I'm sure my younger brother remembers it vividly—the headless chicken that ran straight for him, chasing him around the yard as he screamed at the top of his lungs.

Now I felt like that chicken, running back and forth from one room to the next, fetching medication for David, then a bowl of cereal for the kids, back to the kitchen for a cup of water for Katie, then back again for a rag to clean up spilled water. My days had always been full, but now I had a spectator in my quiet spouse who was unable to help, and needed care himself. Seeing me constantly waiting on young children and trying to keep up with the house, I knew he sometimes hesitated to ask me for help, not wanting to add to my burden. While I thrived on doting on him for the first time in our married life, after a couple of weeks I was also feeling the effects of the extra work. Most likely due to her own anxiety about her daddy, Abby also added to my stress level with her increased demands: following me around the house, whining for attention, and repeatedly asking me to sit next to her on the couch to read books or watch television.

I never left David for more than the hour it took to go into town to the grocery store, taking Abby and Katie with me so they wouldn't bother him while I was gone. One morning, however, I managed to escape the house alone with Katie to run an errand in town. An hour later, in the car on the way home, I purposely passed our turn-off and just kept driving. Katie was completely quiet in the back seat, and I could feel the tension in me disappear as I drove for another fifteen minutes. I wasn't ready to go home and face yet another day of caring for everyone else. I was torn. Part of me wished I could just keep on driving—for an hour, for a few hours, perhaps for an entire day. The other part of me thought about David at home trying to care for a rambunctious toddler, clumsily doing his own feedings, and trying to figure out his medications. I thought about him sitting quietly in his chair, watching me, and delaying his own needs. Of course, I turned the van around and headed home.

When I arrived there, I found David in his chair patiently waiting for me. I dropped my grocery bags at the doorway, went over to him and knelt down, leaning my head against his knees. Taking his hand, I looked up into his eyes and confessed, "I didn't want to come home. I wanted to keep on driving."

"I know. I knew that when you left," he responded quietly as he squeezed my hand. "Thanks for coming back."

• • • •

At some point in those early days of caring for David's needs, I was reminded of how, despite the intensity of caring for a newborn, I still viewed our infants as gifts from God. Similarly, I was finally seeing David as an extraordinary gift in my life. I felt as though it was an honor and a privilege to care for someone I loved. I found, too, that the tender feelings I had been experiencing during his hospital stay were fast becoming feelings of passion and desire.

While common sense would dictate that changing bloody and pus-filled dressings daily might dampen one's desire, I was having the opposite dilemma. I found myself in an almost constant state of arousal and desire for David, my nerve-endings tingling at the slightest touch from him. I couldn't stop touching him: holding his hand as I fell asleep each night, leaning down to kiss the top of his head or caress his arm as I passed the chair where he sat, and more than once, even rubbing his feet with alcohol for the cooling effect it had on hot feet. The first time I did that, he looked startled and asked, "What? Do my feet stink?"

"No, I just love you," I said as I kissed the feet I had never caressed in our twenty-seven years together, even though he had often caressed mine. I'd always thought his feet were funny looking with the second toe that was longer than the big toe, the skinny, crooked other toes, and the bony arches. Now I caressed those same feet and wondered why I had avoided touching them for so many years when, as a young girl, I had thought it was a privilege to rub my father's calloused, tired feet. Back then, my sisters and I would argue over who got to rub Dad's feet with alcohol in the evenings after he'd mowed grass all day.

By three weeks post-op, when it was obvious that David was recovering well, my touches had become blatantly sexual in nature. It didn't take long for me to realize I was being rebuffed. After all, having given birth to and nursed eight babies, I was the queen of rebuffs. I knew all the tricks to avoid sex. It was the ultimate irony that now the tables were turned, and it was I who had the strong desire while David had virtually no libido. I recognized the stiffened back in response to my back rubs at night, the sudden change in topic if I even hinted at David joining me in the shower or the bedroom.

My desire had varied greatly throughout our twenty-seven years together, but David's interest in sex had never waned during that time. It had always been a given in our marriage that he wanted sex. During pregnancies, my sex drive always peaked to an insatiable appetite that had matched his own. After birth, my interest nose-dived until it was almost nonexistent and remained so during the first months of breastfeeding. My desire gradually returned as I started getting longer periods of uninterrupted sleep. During those times when my libido sank to an almost nonexistent level, we'd experienced the typical marital friction resulting from differing levels of sexual appetite, even arguments that escalated to the point of David nastily accusing me of being "frigid" when I rebuffed him one too many times. In all those years, though, David was never the one with a lack of interest, and I'd even joked that if I had the flu, he would have said, "I know what would help you feel better." Given that his constant interest in sex was a set pattern in our marriage, it was quite a shock to see no signs of his libido returning.

Even after David had recovered enough to take short walks with Abby and mown the lawn once, he still did not show any interest in resuming marital relations. His complete lack of desire was unfathomable to me. When we finally did discuss it, David confided that he just had no interest whatsoever. He even had the gall to repeat the same thing I'd occasionally said to him, "It just feels like another chore to me."

This was unprecedented in our marriage. I tried to be understanding, running the litany of possible reasons for his lack of libido through my mind over and over: his recent surgery, the foreboding sense of what was ahead in his treatment, and his worry that I might possibly get pregnant. Still, I couldn't help but take it personally. I was exhausted, wiped out from caring for him, but I still desired him. Why wasn't that being reciprocated? Irrationally, I started wondering if he even loved me anymore. Wasn't I attractive to him? The first time I started crying about his rebuffs, he looked horrified. He'd had no idea I was hurting so much or taking his lack of desire personally. After days of skirting around the issue and more bouts of tears from me, I finally insisted he see our family doctor.

It had occurred to me that his increased blood pressure medication could have something to do with the lack of libido. During his hospitalization, a spike in his blood pressure resulted in the internist on staff tripling his dose of verapamil. No one had altered it since he'd left the hospital, so he was still on triple the dose he'd been on prior the surgery.

I went with David to see our family physician, determined to get my passionate husband back. I thought Dr. Tomas looked slightly amused by my insistence that this situation was not normal for us. He gently countered that perhaps it was a normal reaction with all David had been through. When I pointed out that in twenty-seven years of marriage nothing had affected him this way, not unemployment or his subsequent depression, not my chronic illness or any other stressor, he suggested a change in David's medication. He wanted to put David back on Norvasc, a blood pressure medication he'd been on previously with good results. Since David's blood pressure was not stable on the high dose of verapamil anyway, this seemed like a good idea all around. As we left the office together with a new prescription for a liquid Norvasc that could be put in David's feeding tube, I squeezed David's arm and felt it stiffen under my touch.

"Don't worry," I laughed, "I'm not expecting an instant miracle."

Dr. Tomas had told us it could be days or even weeks before we noticed a difference in David's sex drive if the medication was

73

to blame. We didn't have weeks. Soon David would start his che-motherapy and radiation treatments, and I expected sex would be the last thing on either of our minds. I waited a few days before I broached the subject again, and David finally joined me in the shower. As I rubbed his chest with a soapy sponge, he turned his back to me. Stung, I turned him back around and his eyes met mine as he lamely gestured towards the feeding tube coming from his stomach. Finally, the realization hit me. This was about way more than a low libido. David didn't feel desirable with a tube protrud-ing from his abdomen. I'd told him several times it didn't bother me, but obviously it did him. Instead of telling him as I had been, I attempted to show him how little it mattered to me.

One encounter in the shower didn't solve all our sexual difficul-ties, but it did make me more sensitive to what David was going through emotionally and physically. Still concerned, I decided I would post a question about my spouse's lack of sexual desire on an Internet message board set up for oral cancer patients and their families. When I searched the site, I found I didn't need to post my question. The wife of a man going through a similar treatment had already done so months before. She'd been his caregiver for his first bout with oral cancer and then again since a reoccurrence. He now spent most of his days sleeping in bed, and they hadn't had sex for over two years. I felt guilty and ashamed for my own petty concerns. The majority of the replies to her posting were from the cancer patients themselves, who reiterated that they hadn't been interested in sex either during their cancer treatment. Many said it took months following treatment before they felt a normal desire. One courageous young man in the midst of his treatment suggested that the spouse insist upon physical intimacy for the patient's own good. He wasn't interested either but felt a sense of normalcy when his spouse succeeded in enticing him. Many patients agreed that their large doses of medication probably contributed to a lack of desire.

We wouldn't have a chance to find out if David's libido would return full force on the new medication because we soon had more pressing concerns. Four weeks after his surgery, David began his chemotherapy and radiation treatments.

Chapter Eight

Let the Trials Begin!

During chemo, you're more tired than you've ever been. It's like a cloud passing over the sun, and suddenly you're out. You don't know how you'll answer the door when your groceries are delivered. But you also find that you're stronger than you've ever been. You're clear. Your mortality is at optimal distance, not up so close that it obscures everything else, but close enough to give you depth perception. Previously, it has taken you weeks, months, or years to discover the meaning of an experience. Now it's instantaneous.

—Melissa Bank

Each summer I'd sign up for an adult reading program at our local library. Typically I'd read more than twenty fiction books during the twelve-week period. After David's diagnosis in June of 2006, all I checked out of the library were books pertaining to cancer.

Unlike David, I wanted to know everything I could about what to expect during his treatment. I considered knowledge as power.

The myriad of possible side effects from chemotherapy and radiation boggled my mind. I found myself unable to sleep some nights, possible scenarios of David ending up in a hospital with dehydration or an infection keeping me awake.

David, on the other hand, avoided reading anything at all about cancer, and didn't even care to talk about the subject. Whether this was a form of denial or a coping mechanism didn't really matter; it was what worked for him. I read out loud to David from the books and the websites if I thought the information was pertinent or would be helpful. But the fact that I was immersing myself in cancer information while David practiced an avoidance technique meant my anxiety level about what David's treatment would entail was heightened to extreme proportions. I wanted David to be prepared for anything that might happen, while he wanted to approach his treatment in his own way: meeting each challenge as it came along, if it indeed came up at all. I didn't necessarily understand it, but his approach did have its own merits. There were many things I was worried about that never happened.

Some of the books I read were so helpful that I wanted to own them, so I ordered used copies on the Internet. One book I checked out at the library listed a phone number in the back for any cancer patient or family member to call to receive a complimentary set of three paperbacks. I was amassing a small home library of books on cancer by then, so of course, I called for my free copies. In just a matter of days, they arrived in my mailbox and I pored over them. They were written by an independently wealthy businessman who had survived cancer despite a terminal diagnosis many years before. While his message was uplifting, I had to stop reading after I read the description of his chemotherapy treatments. Even though the room where he'd had his treatments didn't resemble the comfortable room we'd toured where David would be having his, the vivid image of this man and his roommates retching into pans for hours did little to dissipate my fears for David. While we'd been informed that anti-nausea drugs had drastically improved over the past decade, I was still worried about the possibility of Erbitux increasing that nasty side effect of chemotherapy.

The author of another book described chemotherapy as a chemical method of bringing the body as close to death as possible without killing the patient. That did little to dissipate my fears, either. Chemotherapy drugs would destroy many of the important fast-growing cells in David's body along with the cancer cells. It was after reading these books that I started searching the Internet for anything that might lessen the expected side effects of cancer treatment, including natural supplements I could use to help David through his treatment.

I'd also wondered about giving David the herb Echinacea because of its purported immune system boosting qualities. I discovered, however, that even those websites that touted the benefits of Echinacea did not advise using it for cancer patients, precisely because in boosting the already weakened immune system, it could theoretically overtax the compromised system of a patient undergoing cancer treatment.

The first hurdle I encountered as the caregiver of a cancer patient was in feeding David. He'd resumed eating by mouth two weeks following his surgery, so I was making it my goal to see that everything he ate was healthy and full of antioxidants, since I'd read that antioxidants prevent cancer. I'd added green tea and fruit and vegetable juices to our menu and chose the healthiest ingredients for his mostly soft food diet. I knew that halfway into the radiation treatments he would be using the feeding tube again because his throat would become too sore for him to take in enough calories to keep his weight stable.

Initially, I knew David liked the fact that he had lost weight in the hospital with the surgery and that he was continuing to lose more. Like me, he had struggled to lose weight for several years, so it seemed only fair that what he had to go through would have the net benefit of a substantial weight loss. Neither one of us really understood the full implications of Dr. Gordon's warning that he must maintain his weight during treatment. She stated this several times during our initial meetings with her and reiterated it throughout the treatment. She warned that his feeding tube would not be removed until he could maintain his weight on food taken orally. As he became weaker during the treatment, we realized the initial weight loss was a loss in muscle, not fat, and that his body needed a maximum amount of calories to help him fight for his life during treatment. I was dismayed, then, to find that the good and healthy diet I had been giving him after his recovery from surgery was causing him to lose additional weight! By the time he started his treatment in early August, he was already twenty-four pounds lighter than he'd been prior to his surgery. Half of those pounds were lost while he was in the hospital. The subsequent weight loss was due to his inability to consume enough calories once he began eating again. I started to feel like a failure as a caregiver when the pounds continued to drop at each checkup. The nurses encouraged me to give him empty calories, just to keep his weight up.

We would learn in one of our early appointments that Dr. Gordon wanted all of her patients to eliminate green tea, vitamin E, vitamin C, and foods high in antioxidants from their diets during treatment because she believed radiation works best when oxygen is in the tumor environment. According to her, high levels of antioxidants actually worked against the ability of the high energy x-rays to break the strongly attached DNA bonds of the tumor.

In other words, not only was the "healthy diet" I was giving David causing him to lose weight, according to David's radiation oncologist, it wasn't helping the radiation do its job either.

Later, I would discover that cancer experts were split into two camps on the antioxidant issue. One side, like Dr. Gordon, believed that taking antioxidants during cancer treatment could interfere with chemotherapy and radiation by reducing their efficacy, and the other side believed that antioxidants could counter the harmful effects of oxidation in the malignancy process, boosting the effects of therapy and protecting patients from some of the harmful toxic side effects.

I'd become obsessed with David's diet, I realized on one shopping trip when I looked down in my cart at the checkout and saw that the majority of my purchases were for him when normally the contents would have been chosen for my children's benefit. For the first time in years, my shopping and cooking centered on nourishing my husband. There were only a few boxes of macaroni and cheese and frozen pizza snacks thrown in for the kids. I'd already replaced the healthy alternative of frozen chocolate yogurt with high-calorie ice cream. I filled David up on prepared dinners where the meats were as soft as the mashed potatoes, along with puddings, juice with added fiber, canned soups, yogurt, applesauce, high protein breakfast drinks, and other things I knew he could manage to swallow.

David was eating well by the time he began treatment in early August, but we both knew that would change during treatment. On Wednesday, August 9, 2006, David was to receive his first dose of the clinical trial drug, Erbitux. The chemotherapy drug cisplatin would be added to subsequent treatments. Later, we would discover that the cost of Erbitux was between $7000 and $9000 for each infusion. David would receive a total of seven infusions, but as long as he participated in the drug study, the Erbitux would be free. The night before the first dose, I woke David up at 3:00 a.m. to give him Benadryl, then again at 7:00 a.m. He'd have additional allergy drugs given before his treatment because the most common side effect of Erbitux was an allergic reaction.

When we arrived at the oncology office, David had his blood drawn and then saw the oncologist for a quick physical exam. A nurse escorted him to the chemotherapy room, where a couple patients were already receiving treatments. We were greeted enthusiastically by Jenny, a cute nurse with a soft, soothing voice. She helped settle David into a blanket-covered reclining chair, and then wrapped one of his arms with a warm, damp towel to allow the veins to dilate and the skin to soften, since the chemotherapy drugs would be given intravenously through an IV. There were seats nearby for family members or friends. I sat down in the one nearest David's chair and warily eyed the machine that would pump the venomous medication into my husband. Bile rose in my throat as I contemplated the poison coursing through my husband's veins.

Before she started David's IV, Jenny explained that his first infusion would be given slowly over a two-hour period so they could watch for any allergic reactions. Subsequent Erbitux treatments would last less than one hour, but extra fluids and the cisplatin would add another two hours to the treatment.

Jenny carefully checked and rechecked the chart and the bag that contained the medication, punching a code in the machine that would allow the Erbitux to enter David's bloodstream at the speed determined by the doctor. Once the machine was going, I snuck a glance at the other two patients in the room. They both had their IVs coming out of a port in their chests, and they each were accompanied by a female companion. This sight intensified my desire to be with David for his Wednesday treatments. I wouldn't want him to be the only one alone in the room.

One of the patients, a robust, healthy-looking man, was enjoying a large cheeseburger and fries from a Styrofoam container. The woman, who I assumed was his wife, glanced up at me, her eyes moist with unshed tears. She smiled briefly before looking away. Unlike her husband, she seemed to just be picking at her food. I wondered what kind of news they'd heard that day or if she always felt near tears, just like I did. I snuck a glance at the other man, who was extremely thin. He had his eyes closed, and the woman next to him was reading a magazine. A nurse leaned over his chair just then, asking how he was doing. He murmured an answer, "Tired. Just tired." Later, a nurse brought him a large bowl of soup. Seeing the two cancer patients eating as the chemotherapy drugs coursed into their veins was a far cry from the communal retching sessions described in the book I'd recently read!

David's first day of chemotherapy was uneventful, almost anti-climactic after all my worrying and agonizing. For the majority of the two hours we were there, David and I held hands and watched television on the portable set Jenny had wheeled close to us. I delighted in seeing David chuckling at the antics of Jimmie Walker on the *Good Times* series re-run that played. Watching television alone together was just one more thing that had fallen to the wayside in the previous years of raising children. The nurse told us that the most visible side effect from the Erbitux would be an acne-like rash on the face, chest, and shoulder region. In fact, we were told, the medical team rejoiced when they saw it because it meant that the Erbitux was working like it was supposed to.

Directly after the chemo, we headed to the cancer center where David would be receiving his radiation treatments five days a week. At the center, they readjusted the mask he'd been fitted for the week before. He later told me that when they snapped the mask down around his face and shoulders, he had to silently count the minutes in his head to ease the claustrophobia he felt until the treatment was complete.

David's first day of treatment was over, and we headed home. As long as he could manage it, David would be driving himself to the radiation treatments, and as long as I could round up willing babysitters, I would be going with him to his Wednesday chemo-therapy appointments.

Our anxiety over the chemotherapy treatments had abated somewhat by the next Wednesday when David would have the che-motherapy drug cisplatin added to the mix, yet I was still plagued by my imagined visions of him lying in bed, sick and nauseated. In all our years of marriage, I'd only known David to vomit once. I could remember only one other instance when he'd felt so nauseated he'd nearly thrown up, so I had no idea how he would handle constant nausea.

At his second treatment, the medical oncologist gave David a short physical before going over the common side effects of cisplatin, the chemotherapy drug he'd been assigned for six treatments along with the Erbitux. I'd already done my homework on both the drugs cisplatin and docetaxel. The clinical trial would be comparing the survival rates of oral cancer patients taking Erbitux with one of the two chemotherapy drugs. I'd hoped for cisplatin, since it was slightly less likely to cause hair loss than docetaxel and because docetaxel also had the unfortunate tendency to cause eye inflammation. The more serious side effects of both drugs I'd had to gloss over because they scared me too much to even consider. Before treatment could begin, David had to sign a paper noting that he was aware of the fact that cisplatin could cause kidney dysfunction, neuropathy, and hearing loss. He glanced at me briefly before he signed the papers. I knew what he was thinking: these were details I had failed to share with him. When I apologized later for not mentioning those side effects, David just shrugged his shoulders. He understood. He was well aware that any chemotherapy drug could have serious side effects.

Before she concluded her exam, I asked the doctor if she could explain the medications I'd picked up at the pharmacy the day before because I found the directions confusing. "The oncology nurses can do that," was her disappointing response. It seemed to me that the person doing the prescribing should explain the medication. I knew the majority of them were anti-nausea medications, but I had no idea what the others were; all I knew was that they were expensive. When I'd taken the nine prescriptions up to the register without looking at them closely, most of them rang up with co-payments of between $10 and $20 but one rang up at $125.

"Oh, wait, this one must not have been run through his insurance," I said, but the cashier replied that it had, and $125 was the co-pay. I asked her to wait while I went back to the pharmacist to ask why the co-payment was so high.

"Kytril is a top-of-the-line anti-nausea drug," she told me. "That bottle cost $489 before insurance."

What could I say? I wasn't even sure I had the money in my checking account, but I wasn't going to go home and tell David to suffer because we couldn't afford the pills! I wrote out the check for the total $170 and waited until I got out to the van to look at my balance. Sure enough, I had just emptied out our checking account. I opened the bottle and counted just ten pills, not even enough to get David through two weeks of treatment.

•   •   •   •

At David's second treatment, we had expected to see the same two men as the week before, we learned later that they were on a different chemotherapy schedule, not the weekly one David was on. We did see the same woman every week, a fragile looking soul wrapped in a blanket in a corner chair, always wearing a scarf on her head. Neither of us ever spoke to her; she slept through every appointment.

After "our nurse" Jenny set up David's IV, she pulled up a chair to go over the medication chart. I made notes as she succinctly explained which medication to give and when. She explained that because an anti-nausea drug was given in the IV during the treatment, I wouldn't have to start any anti-nausea drugs until the next day. She advised me to give David the drug lorazepam the night after each treatment to reduce anxiety and to help him sleep. She also suggested we stop at a drugstore on the way out of town for Senokot because the anti-nausea drugs were so constipating. We laughed. Constipation seemed the least of our worries. When I told her about the high co-pay on the anti-nausea medication, she checked their office and came back with enough samples of Kytril to use through David's entire treatment, even liquid samples for when he would be unable to swallow.

As we drove home that day, I kept sneaking glances at my husband, anticipating any sign of him not feeling well, but he was fine, just tired. I felt like I was the one who should be taking lorazepam for anxiety since I was nervously watching him, looking for any sign of nausea.

Because we didn't know how David would react to the nine pills he was prescribed, our son Dan gave him a ride to radiation treatments that first week. By Saturday morning, we'd increased the Senokot to twice a day because David was definitely feeling the constipating effects of the anti-nausea medications. To my surprise and relief, what he wasn't feeling was nauseated. At the worst, by Saturday he was burping and hiccupping, experiencing heartburn, and had no appetite. Later, we discovered these symptoms were categorized as nausea under the side effects, but at that point I was just so relieved he wasn't experiencing the terrible vomiting I had imagined.

A pattern of sorts emerged during David's first few weeks of treatment. Wednesday, his chemotherapy treatment day, was actually his best day of the week. He received extra fluids in his IV during his appointment and enjoyed a solid three or four hours of peaceful quiet. He often took naps during the treatments so he felt more rested, too. At home, he spent most of his time upstairs in our bedroom rocking in the rocking chair, trying to read or watch television, but rarely actually sleeping. Since I woke him up earlier on Wednesday, it was easier for him to nap that day. He'd doze off in front of a television while I wrote in the chair next to him. A couple of times he slept so soundly he began snoring loudly, causing me and the nurses to share amused glances across the room. Many times during the treatment he would reach out to take my hand and tell me how happy he was to have me there with him. It was heartrending to see how grateful he was for something as simple as my presence. It became a great honor to share those Wednesday chemotherapy sessions with him. As he faced each treatment with stoicism, my admiration for his emotional strength increased.

David's main complaint was that he felt incredibly full and uncomfortable from constipation. We soon regretted our initial amusement at the nurse's warning. By Thursday or Friday of each week, David would begin to feel uncomfortable because of the constipation that persistently plagued him. By Saturday, he was downright cranky. I pushed the fluids and the Senokot, baked up batches of my never-fail bran muffins, gave him prune juice through his feeding tube (he couldn't stand to drink the stuff), but nothing seemed to work. If he still hadn't gone to the bathroom by Sunday, he would spend the entire day rocking in the rocking chair and complaining with discomfort, avoiding even Dan during his Sunday visits to our home.

During David's early treatment, an e-mail from my friend Barry gave me a glimpse into just how serious that single side effect could be. Barry's brother had lung cancer and was receiving chemotherapy. He ended up in the hospital one weekend, and Barry initially seemed hesitant to explain why. Because he knew that my husband was also a cancer patient, Barry did eventually confide in me the very personal explanation of his brother's hospitalization. Apparently, his brother's constipation had gotten so bad he'd given himself an enema and passed out in the bathroom. His wife found him unconscious on the floor. Because of his weakened immune system from the treatment, the enema had upset the balance in his blood stream and organs, and he became severely dehydrated. This incident served as a reminder to me to not let it get to that point with David, though there were plenty of days he would have appreciated the help of an enema. Usually by Monday morning, David would have had a bowel movement and be feeling much better, only to be facing another week of radiation, chemotherapy, and the constipating drugs following the weekend break.

As if severe constipation weren't enough of a trial, as David's treatment progressed, other side effects of the chemo and radiation became more obvious. By the second week of radiation, the inside of his throat was becoming sensitive and he started to have trouble swallowing most food. Besides the sore throat that was making even talking difficult, David lost his sense of taste and what little he could manage to swallow tasted like cardboard. Before long, all he could eat was Carnation Instant breakfast drinks, scrambled eggs, and the occasional bowl of broth or watery soup, hardly enough calories for a man fighting cancer. In order for him to get adequate nutrition, he had to resort to the feeding tube—the paraphernalia of which we began carting with us to appointments. He'd either have his cans of liquid nutrition during his chemotherapy appointment or in the van on the way to radiation. A hook inside the vehicle was perfect for hanging the bag for the gravity feeding that slowly emptied into his stomach through the tube. Midway through the treatments, he was unable to swallow anything, resorting to complete tube feedings, along with Lortab for the pain.

The "acne-like" rash from the Erbitux added to his discomfort. It looked nothing like any acne I'd ever seen, starting out as a pustule, the pimples soon began oozing, and a crust formed beneath David's beard and down his neck. Combined with the soreness from the radiation on the outside of the neck and the inside of his throat, just turning his head or cleaning his neck was a painful endeavor.

Still, I thought David was handling everything very well until one morning, late into the treatment, when he snapped at me for not understanding something he said. When our son Michael arrived a few minutes later, he had to ask his dad to repeat something, too. David growled at him in a raspy voice. Even his hoarse whisper sounded angry. Michael visibly recoiled, then left the house abruptly without even saying goodbye.

I was stunned that David had gotten angry at Michael for no real reason. He never got mad at Michael. I followed him into the bathroom where he stood before the mirror, washing his neck.

"What's the matter with you?" I demanded. "Why are you being so mean?"

His eyes in the mirror reflected anger. And there was something else. He looked like a wild animal caught in a trap.

"It hurts," he said. "I hurt."

"What hurts?"

"Everything!" he exclaimed despairingly. "Everything hurts. My throat hurts. My neck hurts. I hate this!" He threw down the wash-cloth he'd been using, and I saw it was red with blood.

I realized then that David wasn't just frustrated; he was in pain. I'd really underestimated his pain level up to this point. I gave him a dose of Lortab, which seemed to help within half an hour. Then I went with him to his radiation appointment that afternoon and relayed that morning's bathroom scene to Dr. Gordon. She didn't seem surprised and reminded us that she'd been saying all along that we might have to go to morphine for pain. Besides the mor-phine, she prescribed an antibiotic to fight the skin infection David had developed on his face and neck. She scolded him a little, admonishing him not to wait until the pain was that bad before taking medication.

"You want to keep on top of the pain," she reiterated. I began carrying Lortab with me in my purse in case he needed pain med-ication in between doses of morphine. This marked the end of any solo driving since morphine made him feel uncomfortable behind the wheel.

Considering what I had worried about before David's treat-ment, I still thought things were going fairly smoothly. By the time he'd gotten through three Erbitux treatments, two of the cisplatin treatments, and eight radiation treatments, he still hadn't experi-enced a great deal of nausea, and his main complaint, besides the constipation, was a bone-weary tiredness that sleep didn't relieve. David spent much of his waking hours outside of appointments in the rocking chair in our upstairs bedroom rocking, dozing, or reading. He seemed to need the self-imposed solitude, so I made sure the kids didn't bother him much. We kept busy with our own routines downstairs so that it felt as if he'd gone to work as usual. I'd occasionally check on him, start a feeding, bring him a drink or his medications, but I never stayed upstairs for any length of time or else the kids would begin searching for me. When they did catch me upstairs, I could see how agitated David became, so I encouraged them to come back downstairs with me.

All except for Abby.

Throughout the day, three-year-old Abby would sneak upstairs by herself, plop down at David's feet and either watch television or sit uncharacteristically quietly for an hour, slowly turning the pages of the books from the stack next to her, the books her daddy used to read to her. Sometimes she brought toy animals upstairs and played with them at his feet. I allowed her forays upstairs as long as she wasn't bothering him, because I knew it was good for both of them. Amazingly, Abby seemed to sense what her daddy could tolerate, and she looked forward to spending this time with him. I didn't realize just how important these visits had become to her until one day I heard her crying upstairs. I found her alone in my bedroom, sobbing and pacing back and forth.

"Where is my daddy?" she wailed in a pitiful tone.

She couldn't be consoled, even after I told her he was in the yard. She didn't calm down until I carried her outside so she could see for herself that he was home. After that display of raw emotion, David made a point to inform her anytime he was going outside or would be at a doctor appointment. She was fine as long as she knew where he was, even on the long Wednesdays when we were both gone.

David was handling the treatment well. Abby and the other children were fine with my Wednesday absence. We had everything under control.

Until one Saturday morning when I removed the gauze pad from around David's feeding tube—the sight in front of me made my stomach lurch. The pad was full of green pus. Not just a little, but huge amounts. The pad was soaked with it, and I could see more coming out all around the peg tube. I felt David's forehead but he wasn't feverish. In fact, he said he felt fine, though the area around the tube was sore when I cleaned it. Still, I knew pus was a sign of infection. Though I'd viewed some seepage from that area before, never had I seen such a large amount. I called the local emergency room where a nurse there told me to call the Dubuque emergency room since he was getting his care through them. The nurse at the Dubuque hospital was very concerned.

"People going through cancer treatment are very susceptible to infections and can end up in the hospital very easily. You need to get him to the nearest ER stat," she said.

This was the first time I'd ever heard the word *stat* used outside of the hospital television shows, and it did what it was meant to do: it gave me a real sense of urgency.

I knew about cancer patients and infections. Hadn't I been reading on the cancer message boards about how so many of the patients ended up in the hospital? Wasn't that exactly what I hoped to help David avoid? My anxiety fed off the nurse's anxiety. I didn't need to be told twice. Even though he felt fine, even though he was showing no signs of fever or infection, I told David we had to take him to the emergency room right away. I asked the older children to watch the little ones and hustled David out the door to the nearest hospital.

At the ER, we were put in a room to wait for the doctor on call—not one of the regular doctors on staff, but a stranger to us who was just filling in. He seemed nice enough when he came into the room. He pulled up a chair in front of David and started peppering him with questions: *How do you sleep? How is your appetite? How much do you weigh? What did you weigh when you got married? Do you exercise?* I was becoming agitated, wondering what any of this had to do with pus coming out of his peg tube, but I remained silent.

Then the doctor told David that he was healthier for having lost weight, and that for each ten pounds he lost he would gain a year of life. *What?* He was telling this to a cancer patient? I could remain silent no longer.

"He has been told in no uncertain terms not to be losing weight during his cancer treatment. His doctor is adamant that he not lose any more weight."

The doctor ignored me and continued questioning David. "What medications are you on?"

I started to respond, even though we'd just spent the better part of twenty minutes telling the nurse his list of medications. The doctor interrupted me. "I asked him. I like to hear it from the patient."

"But she's my advocate," David said, slightly panicked. We were both aware that David didn't even know the names of his medications. I pulled the list out of my purse and began reciting the names of the medications again, a list the doctor could have seen on the computer screen if he'd bothered to look. When I realized the doctor was ignoring me, I felt a flash of anger.

Finally, the doctor told David to lie down so he could see the feeding tube. I relaxed a little. At last something would be done about what we were here for instead of the game of "Twenty Questions" the doctor seemed to be playing. For a fleeting second, I wondered if this man really was a doctor. After all, the nurse hadn't come back in with him. He could have been anyone. Maybe he had just donned a white coat and was *playing* a doctor.

The doctor took a look at the feeding tube, flicked it with his finger and said, "It looks fine."

I was incredulous. Of course it looked fine; I had cleaned it up before coming in! I approached and showed him the reddened area, explaining how much pus there had been on the gauze that morning and how it was oozing out of the area before I'd cleaned it.

"Honey," he said, "you just aren't keeping it clean enough. Let me show you how."

He started rubbing the area roughly with the clean, dry gauze I'd put there. He asked what I normally used to clean it. I said I used soap and water, drying the area carefully before applying new gauze.

"You don't need to dry it," he said as he continued rubbing the area with the gauze. "Just clean it like this."

About the time I saw David wincing in pain, I saw blood on the gauze. "I'm not going to rub so hard I make my husband bleed," I retorted.

"It's nothing," he said again, dismissively. "Maybe a stitch came loose."

By now I was just staring at him in disbelief. Was this guy for real? As far as I knew, there were no stitches around a peg tube.

Just then, the nurse came back into the room and the doctor instructed her to apply some antibiotic cream and a new gauze pad on David. Then he pulled off his gloves, leaned against the counter, and started talking again—about politics, war, and Greek gods who put rocks in their mouth so they could talk better.

"Are you going to talk better later?" he asked, and then instead of waiting for an answer, continued his verbose lecture. *The jerk.* Were we supposed to be impressed he was knowledgeable about Greek myths and had an opinion about the Iraq war? What did any of that have to do with the pus-filled gauze issue I brought David in for?

I interrupted his saga to ask him why a nurse in Dubuque would order us to get to an emergency room immediately. He just rolled his eyes, like, *Women.*

"It's nothing. You just need to clean it better," he said for the third time, once again dismissing me and my worries. Then he told the nurse to give us a discharge sheet, handed me the antibiotic cream to use every day, shook David's hand, and had the gall to pat my shoulder on the way out of the room. "Take care of him, sweetie," he said as he left.

I looked at the nurse, waiting for her to tell me the punch line, and that they'd let the maintenance man don a doctor's coat and check patients out occasionally as some big joke. I felt as though I'd been a horrible advocate for David, letting this man rub him raw and dismiss our concerns so airily.

But there was no punch line. Her back was to me as she busied herself with preparing a computer generated discharge sheet. When she handed it to me, I glanced briefly at it. At the bottom of the sheet was a list of instances when I should contact them or bring the patient back in. One of the last sentences jumped out at me, making it my turn to wince: *Contact us immediately if pus is coming out of the peg tube area.*

Chapter Nine

We Get By, With a Little Help from Our Friends

The friend who holds your hand and says the wrong thing is made of dearer stuff than the one who stays away.

—Barbara Kingsolver

Early in 2006, David's family sold some land they had co-owned ever since their father's death in 1991. We received payment for the land in April of 2006. Other than the income tax refunds we got each year that we would apply toward heating bills and large purchases like vehicles, it was the first time in our married life we had some extra money.

The American dream of owning a home had always seemed just out of our reach. The truth was we actually loved the old brick home we were renting and the opportunity to live in the country with our children. It seemed a perfect place to raise our homeschooled children.

Early in our marriage, our college lifestyle and frequent moving was not exactly compatible with owning a home. Later, when we looked into some first-time homebuyer programs, we were disappointed to find out we would have to buy a house within the city limits in order to qualify. And always, there was that specter of our college loan debt looming over us.

So while we initially discussed using the money for a down payment toward home ownership, we decided to first pay off our college loans and all our credit card debt. We also bought a freezer, a stove, and a nice used couch. I was still unable to rationalize buying a new couch while we had little ones who were so hard on furniture. We couldn't bring ourselves to use much money for "fun money," except for making our yearly, one-day trip with the kids to a Chuck E. Cheese restaurant, fifty miles away. Even then, I made sure I had coupons for the pizzas and tokens so we could spend an entire afternoon there for little cost. David and I would laugh as we huddled together in the Chuck E. Cheese photo booth to pose for what we'd begun referring to as our "annual portrait." I enjoyed our trips there as much as the kids did. I sipped pop and wrote, read, or visited with David while our children played for hours.

We put the remaining land sale money in savings, taking an extreme pleasure in the knowledge that we could use it for a down payment on a house later or at least have a cushion of money if something happened.

What happened was cancer.

I figured we could look at the timing of the land sale in one of two ways. We could look at it bitterly as just our luck that the only time we had some extra money something bad would happen and it would all just slip through our fingers. Or, we could look at the land sale as God's way to provide for us during the financial hardship the cancer treatment would cause.

We chose to think of it as God's providence.

David was blessed to have good medical insurance through his place of employment, but there was a yearly deductible he would be responsible for and huge co-payments on some of the medications he needed. Daily trips to Dubuque to visit him in the hospital and later for radiation treatments at a time when gas was nearly three dollars a gallon meant our savings depleted rapidly.

Money, or the lack of it, was to become a constant stressor for David once he felt well enough to start worrying again, but if we hadn't had that cushion to fall back on, it would have been much worse.

It was through friends, and even total strangers, that God showed us how he could provide for our needs. One way was through our oldest son. Even after Dan had moved to Manchester, adding twenty miles to his driving time, he still took David to appointments every other day during the week. By the final week of treatment, we took my sister Denise up on her offer of a ride for David just so we could both get a break.

David's last chemotherapy session was scheduled for September 20 and his final radiation for October 2. While I was thrilled for him at his final chemotherapy treatment, I couldn't help but feel a bittersweet sadness. It would be our last Wednesday alone together. A week later, I decided to take David to his radiation appointment in an attempt to prolong our Wednesday time together.

Before his treatment, the nurse said Dr. Gordon wanted to see him. This was unusual. Normally David saw her after his treatment. While we waited for Dr. Gordon to come into the room, I nervously joked, "Maybe she wants to tell you that you can quit now." He had five treatments remaining and didn't relish coming back over the weekend for his last one.

Dr. Gordon came in the room and took a look inside his throat.

"Have you seen it?" she asked me. When I shook my head, she motioned for me to look. Tears sprang to my eyes as I looked inside my husband's throat for the first time during treatment. It was flaming red, his tongue and mouth peppered with angry-looking sores.

"Mr. Kenyon," Dr. Gordon announced then, "You are done. No more treatments. You've met the criteria for the trial, and you've had enough."

Stunned, we didn't know what to say except thank you.

"You did wonderful," she continued.

I wanted to hug her, but instead we both just shook her hand.

Dr. Gordon warned us David's throat would get worse before it got better, explaining that while the radiation he had already received would not remain in his body, the cells would continue to die up to one month post treatment. Skittish about physical displays of affection and the protocol in regards to boundaries between doctors and patients, I again resisted the urge to hug Dr. Gordon goodbye when we left her office. I regretted my hesitation when I discovered in the vehicle on the way home that David had also resisted the urge to wrap his arms around the doctor who'd felt more like a friend than a medical professional just doing her job. Our instincts turned out to be correct: both David and I would give her the hug she deserved at a follow-up appointment. It wasn't long after his treatment that Dr. Gordon affectionately become "Dr. Suzie," keeping in touch with us even after she left the cancer center and found work elsewhere.

We couldn't wait to inform everyone that David's radiation was complete. We both felt such a huge sense of relief and euphoria that David had gotten through it all. On the way home, I kept telling him how proud I was of him, even though he downplayed his part in the whole process, saying he didn't have any choice but to get through it. I reminded him that Dr. Gordon had said not all her patients were so compliant or hopeful. He did have something to be proud about. He not only did what they asked of him, he'd kept a positive attitude through the majority of his treatment.

We rushed home to tell the kids, who hurrahed in response. The good news posted on my family website was met with celebratory congratulations and evident relief from the siblings who had been an active support for our family. When I called David's brother Keith that night, he was ecstatic, too Everyone who cared about David knew what a long, hard road the treatment had been for him, and the relief we all felt at the conclusion of it was palpable.

The next week flew by. In lieu of the hug I really wanted to give her, I wrote Dr. Gordon a note expressing our appreciation for her care. Contrary to her prediction, David never came to hate her during his treatment. Both David and I hugged her at the first follow-up appointment, unable to withhold our gratitude any longer. She hugged us back, even crying a little as she held onto David.

Each day, I noticed improvement in David. He was still tired, but three weeks after his treatment was complete, he was able to start swallowing some soft foods and his neck looked much better once the infection responded to medication. He attempted short walks, usually with his three-year-old companion. Abby would take his hand and encourage him every step of the way, patiently waiting as he stopped to rest on even the shortest walk. Eventually, he could walk the equivalent distance of a city block down to the barn and back without getting winded. By mid-October, David was feeling better but still couldn't imagine going back to work, even though his sick and vacation pay would soon end. He still had no energy and remained on morphine. Just the short walk from the parking lot to Dr. Gordon's office exhausted him.

"When can I start back to work?" he asked.

"I'd say the end of November at the earliest, and then only part-time," she answered matter-of-factly, then noticed our shocked looks.

"Is that a problem?" she asked. "I can send a social worker down to talk to you if it is."

I asked her to do that, trying to calm the nervous fluttering in my stomach and the rapid beating of my heart. It was times like this I yearned for stronger faith. I wanted to trust that God would take care of us, but I didn't see how he could pull us through an entire month with no income. By the time the social worker came into the room, my stomach was in knots.

After I explained our dilemma, the social worker asked how much money we had on hand.

"Maybe five or six hundred dollars," I answered, doing rapid calculations in my head. I knew we had three hundred in savings and in David's drawer there was at least another two hundred dollars we'd gotten in the mail from concerned friends and family. I was expecting a one hundred dollar check for an article I had published that month, too.

"What are your main bills? The bills that have to be paid?" he asked, writing in a notebook in front of him.

"Our rent. That's $325. That has to be paid for both November and December. Our electric bill is well over two hundred dollars this time of year. That would be due the end of October and the end of November." I said.

Then I suddenly thought of something else. "If David isn't working in November, he will be responsible for paying for the portion of medical insurance his workplace normally pays, and that's over six hundred dollars!"

I felt tears spring to my eyes. We couldn't lose David's health insurance! It didn't take a rocket scientist to figure out we were in big financial trouble.

The social worker continued taking notes, hardly looking up from his notebook.

"So, I've got the rent, the electricity, and the medical insurance. Are those your biggest bills coming up?" he asked.

I wondered how he could sound so calm when I was feeling frantic by now.

"Yes, the rent, the medical insurance, and the electricity are the biggest bills. Then, of course, there is the auto insurance, telephone bill, credit card payments, and food . . . " My voice trailed off.

He looked up then. "Would it help if someone else paid for two months of rent, two months of electricity, and the November insurance premium?"

"Of course that would help," I laughed nervously, wondering what he was getting at. I didn't know anyone who could pay those bills for us.

"Alright then," he continued triumphantly, "have statements detailing those bills sent to my office, and we'll pay them." Then he stood up to shake our hands.

David and I looked at each other in confusion. What had just transpired? The cancer center was going to pay those main bills?

The social worker explained that the center had been left an endowment fund by a wealthy couple who hoped to help people like us during cancer treatment. A maximum of two thousand dollars could be used for each family that qualified to help in paying their bills if they didn't have an income or savings. We shook hands with the social worker and thanked him profusely, in awe at the generosity of complete strangers.

When we got home, I called David's workplace and informed his boss that David's doctor wouldn't allow him to start back to work until late November. He was very understanding. Then I talked to the office manager and told her that the cancer center would be paying for the November premium of the medical insurance and asked her to mail them an invoice with the amount due. She seemed genuinely relieved for us and told me to tell David to concentrate on getting better and not to worry.

By the end of October, David's pain level had decreased enough that he was off the morphine and back to just the Lortab. His neck was still sore, but the rash had disappeared. His energy level had gradually improved but not to a level where I could imagine him resuming his job. Though he enjoyed being at home, it bothered him that he wasn't strong enough to return to work.

Dan was at our house on Halloween when David got a phone call. A short while later, I began getting the children ready for trick-or-treating in town when I noticed how agitated David was. I hurried up the costume preparations, eager to get away from him if he was in one of his moods. He was in the bathroom when I was ready to leave. I opened the door as I called out a goodbye. I was appalled to see him leaning against the counter, sobbing uncontrollably.

"What is it? What's wrong? Are you in pain?"

"I just feel like a failure. I can't work. I feel weak. I don't even feel like myself."

I wrapped my arms around him, feeling a deep sense of fear, noticing, as if for the first time, how thin he'd gotten and how little muscle tone he had. His once broad shoulders were now narrow and bony. By this time, he'd lost almost forty pounds and seemed very fragile to me. For a few seconds, I was terrified by his fragility. In the next instant, I was confused at his emotional weakness. Where was this coming from? David was through the worst. He was on the upswing. He was getting stronger every day. He hadn't cried or lost his strong resolve through this entire ordeal. Then it dawned on me.

"Who was that on the phone?"

"A friend. A friend who felt the need to discuss his retirement plan and how he was all set, financially. And here I am, unable to earn money to take care of my family."

What was that friend thinking, I wondered. *What possessed him to brag about his retirement plan to a man who'd just completed cancer treatment and wasn't able to work?* Right then, watching my strong husband cry, I felt a surge of anger toward that clueless man.

More than that, I was scared. David never cried. I hugged him tighter while he composed himself, and then he apologized.

"Don't apologize. You've been through a lot. You've been through hell. You deserve to cry."

I was so glad Dan was at the house just then. Before I left with the kids, I pulled him aside and told him what I'd just encountered in the bathroom. I saw a flash of fear in Dan's eyes before he patted my arm and reassured me he would talk to his dad while we were gone and the house was quiet.

By early November, it was difficult to imagine David going back to work anytime soon. He was still so weak. It was just as difficult to imagine being able to stretch our money until he could start bringing in a paycheck again. I didn't want David to be worrying, but even with our main bills paid, I didn't know how we were going to make it financially until the beginning of December without an income. I worried. I worried a lot. What I couldn't foresee was what David's coworkers at the nursing home were planning.

On the first Friday in November, the day that David would have gotten a paycheck if he'd had more sick leave, the chaplain from the nursing home dropped by. With a huge smile on her face, she presented David with an envelope, telling him to sit down before he opened it. Inside was more money than David's usual paycheck, some twenty-dollar grocery certificates that his coworkers had turned over from their own Thanksgiving bonus, along with gift cards for a local gas station. David's mouth dropped open and he gave her a big hug. I was near tears myself, humbled by the kindness and generosity of David's coworkers who'd taken up a collection. I wondered if they had any idea what this meant for our family. What they had given him was far more than money. His friends from work had given him the gift of time and peace of mind. Now he, and I, could relax a little. David could take his time getting better before returning to work.

•   •   •   •

In all our years of marriage, David and I hadn't cultivated any lasting friendships with other couples. The "friend" who'd called David after his treatment to talk about his retirement plan could hardly be called a real friend—that was the only contact he'd had with David during his fight with cancer.

David had often expressed envy over my female friendships and my relationship with my sisters. He'd lament his lack of friends outside of our son Dan and a couple family members. I'd never really questioned this, but I'd always felt a little bit guilty about having so much fun with my sisters when we got together, wishing David could have the same pleasure in someone's company.

After his surgery and throughout his treatment, my sisters had continued to offer help in the form of babysitting and gas money. Pat had even given me a cell phone to use while David was in the hospital and gift certificates to her consignment store to help us out financially. She'd stop by the house with little gifts for the kids, a bag of bagels, or other offerings of encouragement.

We both soon discovered that David had more friends than he'd ever imagined. Get-well cards began arriving while David was still in the hospital, continuing throughout his recovery and treatment. One woman from his workplace managed to send a card every single week. Another coworker, who had gone through chemotherapy and radiation herself, made sure he got regular notes of encouragement.

106

One day, while he was still in the hospital, I brought several cards with me on my visit and saw he'd gotten several more sent to his room, along with a large plant from his siblings.

I dropped the stack of cards in his lap and joked, "For someone with no friends, you sure get a lot of cards." He smiled as it dawned on him that maybe some people did care about him and I wasn't the only one with friends.

The outpouring of support for David during treatment and beyond was eye opening for us. Until his illness, David hadn't even realized how many of the people he worked with could be counted as friends. We were humbled by the generosity of others. During David's cancer experience, I came to the realization that I'd become quite cynical over the years, believing there were so few good people in the world anymore. But during David's treatment, we even heard from total strangers who were praying for us, and some had even sent money. They'd heard about our family situation and wanted to help!

Despite all the help we were receiving, reactions to the news of cancer varied greatly. While we felt warmth and love coming from all directions, there remained a void. There were some people we didn't hear from at all, and then, of course, there were those who responded completely inappropriately. David and I really didn't need to be reminded of how often cancer resulted in death.

"Thank you for sharing that," I said to one woman who, after finding out about David's cancer, informed me she'd known several people who had died of the disease recently. She just stared at me blankly.

As for those we didn't hear from, it was difficult to understand why. While David was in the hospital, I attended a book sale where I ran into a former coworker. When I told her about David's cancer, she replied that she'd already heard about it. I was deeply hurt that she hadn't called, written, or even e-mailed with a note of encouragement.

Logically, I knew there were many people who didn't know how to respond to a cancer diagnosis, but our experience made me realize that even an ill-timed or inappropriate response was far better than no response at all. David had one sibling he never heard from—not before surgery or during the months of treatment. Yet even our mailman, Bob, had sent cards and called us. When he'd heard about David's diagnosis, he'd called to tell us the experience would show us who our real friends were. I was glad then that I'd sent Bob cards and a meal when he'd been hospitalized for a hip replacement. At least he knew he could count us among his real friends.

I also noticed that I'd taken to constantly bringing up the subject of David's cancer in public, not just because it was all-consuming in my life but because I'd found that my comments sometimes led to a feeling of kinship with a stranger or acquaintance. I knew our daughter Elizabeth thought I was just trying to elicit sympathy through my frequent remarks about what her dad was going through, but it was far more than that.

She and I talked on the phone daily.

"You mentioned Dad's cancer again, didn't you?" she'd ask me when we discussed our day, and I'd mentioned a particular cashier at the grocery store or someone I'd seen at the library, especially when the incident involved any failings at all on my part. One time I'd forgotten my checkbook. Another time I lamented that I'd had a dozen overdue books at the library. Once, I was speeding and nearly got stopped by a policeman, who shook his finger at me in warning instead. I knew as well as Elizabeth did that if he had actually pulled me over, the tears would be pouring down my face before I even rolled the window down and I would have blubbered something like this:

"My husband has cancer and had to have surgery and couldn't talk or even breathe on his own and was in the hospital for eleven days, and he has to have radiation and chemotherapy, and I have six kids at home and the little one is just three years old, and I'm scared my husband is going to die, and I'm exhausted, and I really don't think I can do all of this anymore."

And if the policeman had ever had cancer or had been a caregiver of a spouse or knew someone close to him who had suffered with some serious illness, he might have let me off without a ticket and maybe shared his own story right then.

Because that is what I was really looking for every time I was too outspoken about our own cancer experience or inappropriately divulged information about David's ongoing personal battle: a connection. So many people had their own story to tell. Yes, I wanted forgiveness for my failings, but even more I wanted that kinship, that acknowledgment of my fragility. Even though I had to appear strong, I often felt terribly weak. I needed to hear that someone else had been through something similar and had come out relatively unscathed on the other side. I wanted those brief moments of real meaning between two strangers: the hand that reached out to cover mine, the quick hug, the moist eyes that would look into my own, or the understanding nod of the head. I wanted a connection with another human being who had traveled this same road, and survived.

Our mailman, Bob, had been correct. During David's cancer treatment, we learned who our real friends were. It wouldn't be soon before we forgot those who had sadly failed us in our time of need. But more importantly, we would never forget the tremendous outpouring of love and generous help by the hands of family, friends, and even strangers.

Chapter Ten

Make It Mean Something

What cancer does is it forces you to focus, to prioritize, and you learn what's important. I mean, I don't sweat the small stuff. . . . And when somebody says you have cancer, you realize it's all small stuff.

—Joel Siegel

Sometime during 2005, the subject of friendship was being discussed on my family's website. I wrote about my longtime friend Mary. We'd met in 1986, when David and I had moved to Iowa City so he could pursue his Master's Degree in Social Work. I was pregnant with Michael, our third child, and my dad had just passed away. I was lonely and felt isolated in an unfamiliar town. Mary arrived at my doorstep, three young children and a plate of homemade chocolate chip cookies in tow. It was Mary who introduced me to a weekly mother's playgroup at her church and my first LaLeche League meeting. It was Mary who walked with me for an hour when my labor started. When we moved from Iowa City a year later, what would become one of the most enduring and rewarding pen-pal relationships of all time began. For nearly twenty years, Mary and I had been writing each other once or twice a week, not even waiting for each other's letters before beginning another one. Besides sharing a love of reading and writing, she and I were kindred spirits when it came to writing letters. Our long, newsy letters could have served as a sort of journal for both of us through all those years of mothering. It was Mary I immediately thought of when the subject of friendship came up.

Then one of my sisters touted her husband as her favored friend. "Butch is my best friend," Pat gushed in her posting, and the heartfelt sentiment brought tears to my eyes. I wanted to think of David that way, I realized with a pang of sadness. Why hadn't I immediately identified him as my best friend? We'd started out our marriage as each other's best allies, writing sappy sentiments about "me and you against the world" in our wedding album. What had happened in those ensuing years that diluted that partnership?

If asked in 2005, I would have blamed the change in our relationship on my husband, a fact I find appalling now. As a starry-eyed newlywed, I'd read Marabel Morgan's *Total Woman*, the Christian woman's marriage guide popular in the 1970s, with admonitions such as this:

> It is only when a woman surrenders her life to her husband, reveres and worships him, and is willing to serve him, that she becomes really beautiful to him. She becomes a priceless jewel, the glory of femininity, his queen. (page 80)

Despite Morgan's popularity in evangelical Christian circles and my sincere desire to be that good Christian wife, I couldn't get past the inane advice she gave to greet my husband at the door wearing nothing but clear plastic wrap. Morgan's well-intended but somewhat lame attempt at imparting the edict of viewing the husband as head of the household didn't go over well with the stubborn woman who'd begun to view her husband as somewhat of a tyrant. Soon after marriage, I'd discovered that my husband had a problem that would create havoc in our relationship. He had a hair-trigger temper when under duress. And by their very nature, children tend to contribute to the stress level in a home, as does a constant struggle to make ends meet.

Research shows that the happiness level in a marriage goes down with the birth of a child and during the newborn stage. As parents of a large family, we never actually left that stage of marriage in our own relationship. There was always a baby or toddler, which inevitably resulted in high levels of noise, whether playing or fighting. It didn't matter if the noise derived from fun or strife, David never handled it well.

The first years of our parenting set the tone of our marriage, and an unhealthy pattern emerged fairly early on. To avoid David's angry outbursts, I learned to deflect the kid's hyperactivity and the stress of caring for young children towards myself. In seeking to "protect" David from stress, I inevitably gave myself additional stress. It began spiraling out of control when we were both students in college with two children. There were times I would take an infant Elizabeth to class with me rather than leave her with her father when he was in a foul mood. For years, except for the times I had to be away for college classes or a paid job, I seldom went anywhere without taking the children. I handled all the bill paying, all the cooking, and most of the cleaning in my misguided attempt to "protect" David from these stressors.

David's temper caused a lot of strife between us, and until he dealt with it directly by seeing a counselor, we employed avoidance techniques that did little for our relationship or for our children's emotional psyches. The children and I never knew where his anger was coming from, but we learned it could be triggered by something as simple as a child spilling a glass of milk or letting a door slam shut. We could be enjoying a family outing one minute, and without warning, one of us would become the target of David's anger the next. I knew it wasn't fair for our children to be growing up with the uncertainty of a parent's uncontrolled rage, but it was years before I insisted David seek help with his anger, long enough that our family dynamics were, at best, damaged, and at worst, dysfunctional.

Once I became a full-time stay-at-home mom in 1986, I continued to deny my own needs in an attempt to keep the stress off David. David contributed to the problem by allowing, or maybe even encouraging, me to take the hard road in our parenting, the one that involved constant care of the children. Even after David started seeing a counselor in 1994, gradually learning tactics to manage anger, the unhealthy patterns in our marriage didn't change. They seemed set in stone. While I should have shown respect for my husband, instead I berated him in front of the children, contributing to their lack of respect for him. Even during periods of relative stability and geniality in our marriage (and there were still many of those), that undercurrent of anger over David's previous mistreatment remained within me. I'd wrapped myself in a cloak of resentment that served to separate me from the husband, whose real desire was simply to be loved.

Instead of dealing with our relationship directly, I found a way to keep myself sane by funneling my creative energy into writing, eventually working for a newspaper that paid me to leave the house occasionally to cover school board and city council meetings. When I was pregnant with Matthew in 1993, I started homeschooling. I abandoned the newspaper job after several attempts of taking a nursing infant with me to meetings, but continued to write as a mental escape from intensive mothering and an outlet for my creativity. By the time Emily was born in 1996, I'd had my first book published and was writing regularly for magazines, a pastime that may very well have saved my sanity.

My feeble attempts to get some much-needed time alone resulted in more strained relations between David and me. While David occasionally half-heartedly offered to watch the children while I went shopping or took a walk, he also tended to sabotage my efforts before I even reached the door.

"Go then. Just go!" he might snap at me if I pleaded for some time alone, his loud voice calling attention to me just as I was attempting to sneak out the back door to avoid confrontation with a clinging toddler. Whichever toddler it was at the time would come running, screeching, "Mommy, Mommy, me go, too!" Glaring in David's direction, I'd feel the air rush out of me and I'd give up and just stay home, resenting David and the lifestyle of my own making that left me feeling trapped. I knew the situation had gotten out of hand when I began looking forward to giving birth just so that I could spend some time alone in the hospital.

I was miserable, feeling powerless to change the set patterns in our marriage. Instead, I regularly felt a surge of resentment rise up inside me. I usually managed to control my anger with the kids, but there were many venomous outbursts targeted at David.

"I feel so angry. I don't know where this is coming from," I confessed during a counseling session. By 1994, David and I had turned to occasional visits with a Christian marriage counselor. The fact that a baby or toddler inevitably attended the sessions with us might have been a clue as to one of the major problems in our relationship, yet none of the counselors we saw suggested we come alone. Perhaps they sensed I wouldn't have come at all if I hadn't been allowed to bring whichever child was our youngest at the time.

"Yes, you do. You know where it is coming from," that particular counselor countered. I searched deep inside myself and was ashamed for being so angry at a husband who was trying so hard to be a better person.

"Sometimes when one partner gets help with their anger, the other partner starts to have problems with anger themselves, in response to the patterns of their marriage changing," the counselor continued.

I shrugged this observation off. It wasn't *me* with the anger issues, I though*t*. *I'm* not the one with the problem. I doggedly continued to deflect stressful situations toward myself, never sharing budget dilemmas or concerns about the children with David. I never let him be a true partner in our marriage because I didn't trust his reaction to stressful situations, even though he'd become a different father and husband than he had been for the first fifteen years of our marriage.

David may have gotten his anger under control, but I'd rationalized my antagonistic behavior with the idea that David didn't deserve respect because of those years he'd lashed out at his family with unreasonable anger. His temper had continued to come between us, even after it was under control.

It wasn't until I was driving with my daughter Elizabeth to visit her dad in the hospital following his cancer surgery that it dawned on me. For the first time in many years, I felt no resentment or anger toward David.

"It's gone," I informed Elizabeth in amazement. "I've finally let go of all that anger and resentment I've been holding on to."

She didn't need me to explain. Since her marriage, Elizabeth and I had discussed the unhealthy patterns marriages can get into. She'd dissected our marriage along with me in our conversations. I couldn't explain all the patterns or my inability to change them, either. Tears streaked down my cheeks as I realized how wonderful it was to fall back in love with my husband and to feel hope and joy in a relationship again.

"I'm glad," Elizabeth said softly, "I used to feel sorry for Dad sometimes when you were mean to him. I know he wasn't always nice to you, but he seemed so sad and alone in the kitchen doing dishes after you'd yell at him." It struck me then how perceptive children can be while the adults around them demonstrate relationships they would never wish upon anyone, least of all their own children.

Since David's cancer diagnosis, we'd had a reprieve from even the slightest argument, and I found it refreshing and amazing. After all we'd been through, I couldn't even imagine being angry with him and I thought he felt the same way. I wondered if there was some truth to the simplistic advice to treat your husband right to invoke positive changes in your marriage. I'd never treated David as well as I did after his cancer diagnosis. I truly cared for him physically and emotionally. I'd cherished him, and he'd reacted with a similar tenderness toward me. What if the secret to a successful marriage was as simple as that?

In the face of losing David, I'd finally let go of all the emotional baggage I'd lugged around for years in our marriage, only wanting to make him happy. Had I come full circle in our relationship—worshiping, revering, and serving my husband as Marabel Morgan had advised in her 70s tome—or was I simply forming a real partnership with my spouse?

Since David's cancer diagnosis in June, we hadn't even exchanged strong words. That changed one day late in October.

I usually got up before anyone else, spending a quiet hour to myself before any of the children rose. This morning, however, I'd slept in, and David was already awake when I got up. Waiting for him to get out of the bathroom, I put on the teapot, cleaned off the kitchen counters, and threw what I thought was the dish cloth from the day before into the basket by the basement door for the laundry. Then I went into the office to do some work on the computer.

I was waiting for the computer to boot up when David's angry face appeared around the corner of the doorway.

"You threw the dishcloth away without even asking me if I'd been using it. You always do things like that," he hissed in an all-too-familiar voice, and I cringed, my hands stilled above the keyboard.

We hadn't argued in months, and now he was angry about a dishcloth?

"I thought it was from yesterday," I sputtered defensively, but he'd already disappeared.

Hot tears rolled down my cheeks, a lump forming in my throat. I clutched my hands together in my lap, feeling them start to shake. The stab of hurt was deep. How could he be so angry about something so stupid? Then my hurt quickly worked up to a frenzy of anger. I was furious! How dare he get angry at me after all I had done for him the past months!

Just then his contrite face appeared at the doorway again.

"I'm sorry," he said. "My neck hurts so badly today. I didn't mean to snap at you."

I appreciated his apology, but I couldn't meet his eyes, I was still so hurt and confused. I could barely catch my breath, and my chest felt uncomfortably full of the old resentment I thought I'd abandoned in July.

I followed David to the kitchen and silently and efficiently measured out the pain medication, adding it to his feeding tube, still not meeting his eyes. I couldn't. His comments hurt too much, and I couldn't bear the thought that we might be reverting to our old patterns. David was quiet, too, but I didn't know if that was because he was embarrassed at his outburst or in pain. One of the hallmarks of his unreasonable anger had always been that he'd seem to forget hurling the angry words as soon as he'd said them. Never before contrite, he'd always been genuinely surprised at my reaction and shocked when I'd repeat (usually word for word because I didn't forget easily) the awful words he'd hurled at me in anger.

But this time he apologized immediately, I reminded myself.

I approached David upstairs a short time later as he prepared his own feeding. He apologized again. So he did remember. This was not one of our old patterns. I sat down on the bed across from him and looked directly in his eyes.

"Let's make sure this cancer means something in our life." I said gently.

"What do you mean?"

This was very important to me. I wanted cancer to have changed both of us and our marriage, but I didn't want David to feel like I was blaming him for all the problems we'd had. We both agreed we loved each other more now than ever. I never wanted to fall back into an unhealthy pattern of blaming and resentment. I chose my words very carefully.

"Let's not regress in our newfound relationship and go back to our pre-cancer life, arguing about stupid things that don't matter in the larger scheme of things. If we've learned anything from this experience, let's have learned what is really important in life, and it isn't dirty dishcloths."

David had the grace to blush at this, and he took my hands in his as I continued. "Let's make this the start of our new life together, a better life. Let's treat each other and the kids better. I want our marriage to be stronger. I love you so much. I cherish you. Please don't fall back into your old habits, and I promise to never forget to appreciate you. Make cancer mean something. Don't let all that you've gone through be for nothing."

He smiled then and pulled me to him. "We'll be like butterflies in our new life," he said, and we both laughed.

• • • •

David started back to work part-time the day before Thanksgiving. He still seemed so fragile and weak to me. It wasn't amusing that if a jar needed opening in our house, David now handed it to me to loosen the lid, instead of the other way around. I was seriously concerned about his ability to work. It comforted me to have our son-in-law, Ben, working there. I knew he would keep an eye on David and not let him overdo it. His boss, Doug, promised to do the same.

On his first day back, I hugged David goodbye and the children gathered around him for their hugs, too. With a pang, I felt his thin shoulders beneath my hands, and I saw the look of trepidation in his eyes. We clung to each other a little too long until I realized I wasn't helping him by my clinging. As I looked into my husband's eyes that morning, I realized that this wasn't just nervousness about returning to work—David genuinely didn't want to leave us. Despite their loud boisterousness and our frenetic pace, David had learned to enjoy being around me and the children every day. Despite the noisy house, the bickering amongst the children, and the ongoing messes, he was going to miss us, even for the four or five hours he'd be gone working. It was a bittersweet moment. We were glad David was well enough to return to work, but we both wished he could stay home. Abby kissed him several times, returning to the playroom only to run out the door after him for "one more hug." I yearned to do the same.

It took me several weeks to abandon the protective, mothering feeling I had over David's welfare. As promised, Ben and Doug did keep an eye on David, not pushing him too much and finding light work duty for him with frequent breaks. I provided high protein snack bars for David to eat and reminded him to listen to his body as Dr. Gordon had advised. From other cancer patients, we'd learned that it was common to need one month of recovery for each week of treatment. We didn't expect, then, for David to feel like himself until late March at the earliest. He still coughed and choked as he ate, so he arranged to have his meals alone in the break room.

As December and our first post-cancer Christmas approached, David's stamina increased, as did his work hours. We gradually got used to having David gone more, but we still loved it when he had a day off.

Elizabeth had confided in me that she wanted to make this Christmas special for David after all he'd been through. I felt the same. Because David couldn't get enough of all the *Seinfeld* DVDs that Dan had brought him during his treatment, Elizabeth decided on a gift that was related to the show. She found a set of Seinfeld coffee mugs through an online auction site and bought them for David. Dan had purchased a humidifier to help keep his dad's mouth and throat moist at night. By early December, with only three weeks until Christmas, I still hadn't come up with a gift that would top either of those in special meaning. Around that time, my friend Jacki reminded me of her offer to make a scrapbook for David. Since she was a Creative Memories consultant, I knew the scrapbook would be beautiful. I'd tried scrapbooking once and was a dismal failure at it—wanting to hurry up and finish it, not relishing the incredible time and effort it took to produce one simple page. The idea of a scrapbook representing our life together appealed to me as a meaningful gift for this first post-cancer Christmas, so I finally took Jacki up on the offer.

I spent hours while David was at work, sorting through boxes and boxes of photos. The piles of snapshots I spread out around me told our story in a surprisingly accurate way. Choosing photos from our dating days and early marriage was easy. They were plentiful and we looked genuinely happy. Through the span of years, however, photos of us together were fewer, and by the time I got to the single photo of us at our 25th anniversary party, I paused and reflected on the painful truth. Guests had requested the photo-op where we mugged for the cameras, feeding each other cake. I studied the picture. I recognized my fake smile, the frustration that had become a constant in my eyes. When Elizabeth had told me of her plans for an anniversary party, I hadn't relished being a hostess when I had an infant to care for, and my fears were well-founded. I'd spent the better part of an hour walking around outside in the hot sun with a cranky Abby strapped to me in the backpack, trying to calm her down and get her to sleep. By the time I returned to the party, I was hot, sweaty, and extremely frustrated.

I hesitated including the anniversary photograph but then decided I needed it in there as a constant reminder of what can happen to a marriage that is not nurtured. After labeling the snapshots I'd chosen with sticky notes, I mailed a huge Priority mailer of photos representing our dating days, marriage, and parenting to my friend, and eagerly awaited the final product, getting more and more excited as Christmas Day approached. Two days before Christmas, the scrapbook arrived. Jacki had outdone herself, carefully cutting and arranging the photos in an artful array on the pages. I paged through it several times, smiling to myself. It was exactly what I wanted, a beautiful array of photos that represented the last 27 years. I wrapped the scrapbook carefully, and on Christmas Eve, I hid it beneath all the other gifts under the tree to make sure it would be the last gift David opened.

Christmas of 2006 will always be a magical one in my memories: a Christmas that should have been sparse, considering all we'd gone through and how little money we had by then. Instead, there were many wonderful gifts under the tree. I'd done a large portion of our Christmas shopping early in the spring before David's cancer diagnosis when Amazon.com and Toys "R" Us had a tremendous online sale of toys. I'd gotten several thirty-dollar toys for less than six dollars, with free shipping. The chaplain at the nursing home where David worked had also surprised us in mid-December with large gift bags full of carefully chosen gifts for each of our children and candy we used to fill their stockings. Miriam, a woman from our church, had invited us to peruse the stock of donations in her basement, where I'd discovered warm mittens, socks, and some other things the kids needed.

And, if we had ever doubted God's providence, the Christmas season was brought home to us in the form of two greeting cards that arrived in our mailbox. One was signed, *Jesus* and contained a grocery store gift certificate. The other was simply signed, *Someone who cares* and contained three one-hundred-dollar bills. We were horrified and in awe at the same time. Who did we know that would trust the mail system so blithely, and who could afford such a generous gift? We looked for clues in the masculine signature and the postal mark, but all of the mail from my family and our close friends went through the same Cedar Rapids office. Trying to guess who sent it was a fruitless endeavor but one that prompted us to think positively about each and every person we came into contact with during that Christmas season. Perhaps someone we felt hadn't been very helpful had actually chosen this anonymous way to show their support.

I love Christmas mornings in a house full of children. I'm almost always the first one awake, either waiting in bed until I hear the first stirrings of little feet or sitting in the dark living room brightened only by the light of the Christmas tree, sipping a cup of hot coffee while waiting for children to stumble sleepily down the stairs, their eyes widening when they see the bounty underneath the tree. Our children are always allowed to go through their stockings first, without waiting for their siblings or their parents. My reward for the weeks of preparation is in their faces as I watch them go through the stockings and open their gifts. Because of my year-round shopping and my clearance purchases, combined with garage sale finds and refund premiums, I have always managed to give a bounty of gifts that one morning—a little bit of magic for a family financially strapped the rest of the year.

That year was no exception, particularly because of the generosity of others. After the children opened their gifts and David and I were surrounded by gifts, too, the package that held the scrapbook was handed to David to open. The room got quiet, and we all watched David expectantly. Even the little ones knew that this was a special gift from Mommy to Daddy. David ripped open the paper, revealing the soft tan cover of the scrapbook.

"What is this?" he asked quizzically, his eyes meeting mine. I'd given him several books this year, but he sensed this was something different.

"I wanted to give you something special, after all you've been through," I said as he opened the book and started looking at the photos. I watched his expression soften as he turned the pages. He realized what this gift was: a pictorial history of our life together. His eyes widened in disbelief.

"Did you make this?" he said in awe, and I knew he truly recognized the beauty in the book.

"My friend Jacki did. I chose the pictures."

He spent several more minutes thumbing through it and then he looked up, and I saw the genuine pleasure in his eyes.

"It's wonderful, thank you so much," he said and I smiled back at him. What he left unsaid, what the look between us meant, was that the scrapbook represented our old life, the life before cancer, and our new life was just beginning. We were both excited about our future together—as best friends.

Chapter Eleven

Life After Cancer

Loving someone is about giving, not receiving.

—**Nicholas Sparks**

I once read a book by a woman who'd lamented that she'd spent three entire years of her adult life nursing her three babies, and that was enough for anyone. I laughed out loud. I'd spent three years nursing just one of my eight children. Altogether, I'd spent a total of eighteen years of my adult life nursing infants and toddlers.

While I certainly didn't regret my choice to breastfeed my children or their subsequent robust health, by the time Abby weaned completely, there was no doubt that the sheer number of years I was on call 24/7 had drained me in many ways. I had to admit that my reason for adopting the "family bed" concept had more to do with exhaustion than anything else. We'd fallen into it by default after experiencing many sleep-deprived months with Michael, our third baby. The previous two had slept in cribs most of the night, just waking up occasionally for night-time nursing in a rocking chair. Michael, an angelic baby by day, transformed into a sleepless terror by night. I was lucky if he slept in his crib a total of two hours. Only rocking calmed my midnight beast. I literally rocked one chair to pieces. There were times in the middle of the night when I would give up completely on sleep and strap Michael in the car seat, heading to the nearest 24-hour restaurant. I'd sip decaf coffee and study for college exams while he ate slices of buttery toast. Other patrons would look quizzically at the blonde-haired toddler awake at midnight, and Michael would wave and smile cheerfully at them.

I craved sleep and stumbled around in a daze during the day. Holding my crying child at night in the chair, I would sob in exhaustion and frustration. After Rachel was born, I wasn't about to lose any precious sleep, so she just slept with me. From that point on, each of our children slept in our bed from birth until they were weaned to a toddler bed. While I'd enjoyed an extraordinary bond with my nursing babies that extended into the nighttime hours, it was likely my mothering style had also contributed to, or at least been a symptom of, the deterioration of my relationship with my spouse. This poem I'd written in 2005 reflected my conflicted feelings:

Family Bed

Mattress strewn with blankets,
legs, and small bodies.
My husband displaced,
sleeping on the floor.
I've been in a cock-fight,
and the other bird won.
Hair a tangled mess,
shirt around my neck,
instant access for nursing.
Bones ache from
sleeping on the edge.
Before I had children
I thought bed was a place
to make love.
Not war.

The line "My husband, displaced" spoke an uncomfortable truth I hadn't been ready to admit to until during David's cancer treatment when I saw how easily my children had adapted to my occasional absence as I spent time caring for their father. In those twenty-seven years of very intense mothering, my husband had, indeed, become displaced in our bed and our marriage.

The feelings of love and passion that had been reignited in me during David's hospital stay had not dissipated. If anything, they had deepened during our journey together through his treatments. Our relationship felt new and exciting. It was as though we truly had come out of a cocoon and become butterflies. Both of us felt it, and we were in awe of the difference in our marriage and relationship post-cancer. I sometimes had to resist the urge to herald the love I felt for David in a public place. I wanted to shout out, "I love my husband!" in the midst of a crowded mall. We held hands wherever we went. David kissed me in the kitchen and followed me to the basement when I did laundry. I'd laugh lustily as he pressed me up against the washer and threaten to "ravish me." It was corny for two old folks, but it was wonderful.

Despite this newfound joy in our relationship, by February of 2007, I was experiencing an extreme anxiety that affected my daily life. David was back to work full-time and doing very well. My stint as a caregiver was completed, so I should have been feeling a sense of relief. Instead, I found myself feeling anxious all the time. The children bore the brunt of my anxiety when I'd snap at them over the least little infraction. Katie and Abby were acting up more frequently, likely in a delayed response to their father's illness and their mother's lack of attention. When they acted out in a public place, I'd feel a desperate sense of urgency to just leave, even if I had a cart full of groceries to pay for. My anger arrived full-force, quickly, and with such fierce waves I sometimes felt like my head was going to explode. I had no idea what was the matter with me. I never acted this way with David, but he saw glimpses of my frustration and continually asked if there was something he could do to help me.

Rather than see a doctor, I attempted to figure it for out myself. Was it related to my constant, underlying worry that David's cancer would return? I went with David to each of his CT scans and doctor's appointments, so there was that regular reminder of the reality that oral cancer can return. Or could it be a hormonal imbalance after weaning Abby, along with perimenopause symptoms I'd begun experiencing? I wondered, too, if it might also be a kind of post-traumatic stress disorder brought on by the cessation of David's need for me after months of intensive caregiving. Instead of experiencing relief at the prospect of David becoming independent of my care, I inexplicably felt some disappointment that he didn't need me as much.

Or was it simply a combination of all of these factors? I tried writing and journaling more, getting up earlier and spending that quiet time reflecting on our experience and what it had meant for our marriage. The early morning writing sessions seemed to help me emotionally, but physically I was still a mess. I was tired, overweight, and out of shape.

When I finally confided in David how I was feeling, he suggested I begin taking regular walks to take a break from children and get some fresh air and exercise. I tried, but the country roads were often icy, muddy, or downright dangerous in the dark before children were awake. Once Abby was awake, I faced the added frustration of prying myself away from her increased clinginess.

When David urged me to call the gym in town, I was incredulous. Beauty parlors and gyms were an indulgence I wasn't used to. David's concern for me overrode his worry about the sad state of our budget. After a few more aborted attempts at taking a walk on the gravel road, I was convinced that he was right, and the only exercise program that would really work for me was one in which I left my house to do it. I called both the recreation center and a woman's gym, but the monthly fees for one and the sign-up fees for the other were exorbitant, so I reluctantly gave up on the idea. That is, until a pamphlet from the Dove company arrived in my mailbox in early March. Dove was teaming up with the Curves Company and offering three months free for new members with a proof of purchase for one of their new products, a line of merchandise targeted at older women. A single proof of purchase? I'd just bought fourteen of their Pro-Age face cleansers with high-value coupons and a special Walgreens sale! When I stopped in the Curves gym, the owner told me they were also offering a special half-price registration fee that week. The price of a membership was finally within my reach. So, in March of 2007, with slight trepidation, I joined Curves and, for the first time in a long time, took a huge step towards taking care of myself.

I immediately noticed a release in the anxiety that had become a constant in my life, and gradually noticed an improvement in my energy level as I built up muscle tone. With a regular break from childcare, my angry outbursts noticeably diminished, and both the children and my husband appreciated the difference—the children with a calmer mother, and my husband with a more balanced wife who initiated more romps in the basement. I couldn't help but feel guilty at the indulgence, but it would be almost four months before I would have to pay anything towards my membership again, and David was so happy to see the change in his wife, he more than likely would have been willing to pay full price for it.

As June and our wedding anniversary approached, Elizabeth reminded me of her offer to watch the kids overnight while her Dad and I went someplace to celebrate twenty-eight years of marriage.

We'd never gone on an overnight trip away from children. In fact, one time, when we'd had only four children, David had won a weekend trip. Although we'd had my mother watch the two older children in our home, we'd taken the two youngest with us. At the time, I couldn't bear the thought of leaving the two parentless for an entire weekend. Except for my hospital stays after a birth, I'd never been away from my children overnight. I wasn't completely comfortable with the idea of leaving the children overnight, despite my newfound enjoyment in my spouse. When I saw David's eagerness to be alone with me, I reconsidered.

Abby was almost four years old, and with a trustworthy babysitter offering her services, I allowed myself to consider the prospect, discovering that I not only liked it, but I relished the idea of being alone with my newfound lover. Despite our renewed relationship, up until that point, all our "dates" consisted of doctor's appointments and medical procedures. We both liked the idea of renting a hotel room in the town where we had met, gone to college, and raised our first three children. I went online and gazed at the lovely rooms in the historic downtown Blackhawk Hotel in Cedar Falls, getting more and more excited. When I saw the prices, my heart sank. How could we afford even a one-night stay? In the next instant, I considered all David had been through and how much he meant to me. I thought about twenty-eight years of marriage without even one couple's night away. I was determined to find a way.

In cleaning closets a few days later, I came across my wedding dress stored inside a plastic bag. A slow smile spread across my face as inspiration hit. In 1979, I'd bought the ivory lace Jessica McClintock Gunne Sax dress at a discount because it was missing two back buttons at the collar. If I remembered correctly, I'd paid less than fifty dollars for it back then. As much as I hated to view it that way, it was now considered an authentic *vintage* dress. It had hung in my closet for nearly twenty-eight years. It was a size nine and had been tight on me then, eight babies and too many pounds ago. I'd had the romantic notion that I'd fit into it again someday or my daughters would wear it on their wedding days. Who was I kidding? I wasn't going to wear a size nine anytime soon, and none of my daughters found it even remotely appealing. Since this trip would herald our new life after cancer and we'd never taken a real honeymoon, we'd both taken to describing our anniversary plans as our "honeymoon." I decided to begin a "honeymoon fund," and the dress would be a casualty in my private fundraising efforts.

The dress sold for forty dollars, a nice beginning to the stash of money I was stowing in my sock drawer. From then on, every time I saved money at the grocery store with coupons, I put the savings in my drawer, sometimes adding as much as twenty dollars after a shopping trip. It wasn't long before I had enough saved to pay for the Junior Deluxe Honeymoon Suite at the Blackhawk Hotel in Cedar Falls where I'd made reservations. Then, for several weeks beforehand, I alternated between feelings of extreme excitement and anticipation and those of concern over Abby. I knew Elizabeth could handle just about any situation that would come up, but I wondered how Abby would sleep without being able to climb in next to me during the night. We "practiced" having her fall asleep next to Emily on the bed and talked about her upcoming sleepover for several weeks until she started to get excited about the idea herself.

On the morning of May 31, after dropping the three little girls off at Elizabeth's, David and I headed for Cedar Falls. I felt like a schoolgirl on her first date, heady with excitement. Dan had given us a card before we left, and I opened it on the way. He'd given us twenty dollars and admonished us to go somewhere special. We laughed. He knew us well and realized without his gift we might end up eating our evening meal someplace like a Hy-Vee deli, which is exactly where we stopped for lunch.

The first place we stopped when we arrived in Cedar Falls was the Chuck E. Cheese's restaurant where we'd celebrated several birthdays when we lived there. Holding hands, we sheepishly entered the arena of family fun—for the first time without children. Our plan was to get our picture taken in the photo booth and get out of there. From the entrance, we scanned the room, but didn't see the booth anywhere. When a young girl came over to let us in, I explained that we were celebrating our anniversary and wanted a picture taken in their photo booth to mark the occasion. She laughed but told us they didn't have the picture-taking machine, and the nearest one was in Cedar Rapids. As giddy as we felt, for a few brief seconds I think we actually considered the long drive to that Chuck E. Cheese's, more than sixty miles away. But we had more pressing plans that evening, including a book sale at the nearby Waterloo library.

The fact that I had a husband who understood and encouraged my obsession with books meant the world to me. The idea that he was willing to accompany me to a book sale during what was meant to be a "honeymoon" meant even more. But then, David had always encouraged me to pursue my twin passions of reading and writing, claiming that it was my mind that attracted me to him in the first place, though I was still convinced it was my frugality and the free pie and BLT from our initial date.

When we checked in at the hotel that afternoon, David smiled as I pulled out the wad of bills I'd managed to save for the occasion. We shared an amused glance at the face of the desk clerk who seemed unsure of what to do with the stack of cash. Neither one of us was worldly enough to realize ahead of time that a credit card would need to be on file. I stifled back a giggle as I handed over the card, guessing from her smirk what must have been going through the clerk's mind.

"I'm sure those two country hicks weren't married," David and I imagined her saying later. "Or at least not to each other."

As we ascended the steps to our room, we held hands and gazed at the plush carpet and the lovely antique decorations on the walls. We were both aware that we were definitely way out of our element in this luxurious setting, but it was fun to share in that knowledge. It was me and David against the world again, the couple that would be "forever in blue jeans," just as our favorite Neil Diamond song proclaimed.

The room didn't disappoint, with the genuine antique furniture and fine linens, and our main interest, the big Jacuzzi tub. After dropping our suitcase on the bed, David headed to the bathroom while I attempted to set a romantic mood. I discovered plush bathrobes in the closet and lay them out close to the Jacuzzi tub. I turned the lamp down low and looked in my overnight case for the fragrant body wash I'd purchased for the occasion. In the semi-darkness, I turned on the water and added just a small capful as the warm water filled the tub. Ironically, I felt shy and virginal with my husband of twenty-eight years, and I wanted bubbles to be covering my naked form when he came out of the bathroom. I removed my clothing and gingerly entered the big tub, fumbling clumsily with the knobs until I was able to turn on the jets. Bubbles immediately appeared, covering me. I turned off the jets and waited for David.

I couldn't read the expression on his face when he came out of the bathroom, but I motioned him to join me in the tub as I turned the jet sprayers back on. A few minutes later, we faced each other in the warm bubbles and I felt a delicious thrill, rubbing my feet along his legs and then leaning back to relax. David did the same. *Ah, this is the life*, I thought. I closed my eyes for several moments and when

I opened them, a huge mountain of bubbles nearly obstructed my view of David, whose eyes were still closed.

I swiped frantically at the bubbles, to no avail, barely able to see the top of David's head. I turned off the jets, cleared my throat, and in a small voice said to my now invisible husband, "I guess you aren't supposed to use body wash in a Jacuzzi tub."

David just snorted in answer, and I had to laugh. With some difficulty, I scrambled to my knees and managed to get out of the tub. Still laughing, I toweled off and put on one of the robes. David had a harder time of it, slipping and sliding as he tried to get out, and I finally had to help him out, choking back laughter as I did so. By the time he got out of the tub, I was laughing hysterically. It was an auspicious start to our "romantic" night away. Our futile efforts to get rid of the bubbles only added to the amusement. Once we turned on the overhead lights I wryly noted the small sign warning visitors not to use their own soaps in the tub.

When we left the hotel room a short while later, the tub was fairly clean of bubbles. After a productive book sale that netted us six boxes of books, we enjoyed a delicious, candle-lit pasta meal and then headed back to the hotel room.

We got very little sleep that night, not due to the passion between the sheets, though there was certainly some of that. Instead, we found ourselves tossing and turning in the strange bed, listening to the unfamiliar street noises until 3:00 a.m., when I sighed and suggested we trade sides to see if that would help. It did, and we finally fell into an exhausted stupor just three hours before we simultaneously woke up, smiling at each other. Bleary-eyed, we sat in the hotel lobby at 7:00 a.m., drinking cups of hot coffee and imbibing the free continental breakfast. Reading the local newspaper, I noted out loud that there was a garage sale that day that advertised educational materials. David just looked at me and laughed. He knew that look in my eyes, and it had nothing to do with a repeat of last night's lovemaking and everything to do with my insatiable appetite for good books and good deals. I knew we'd be visiting that garage sale before we left town.

Sure enough, when we left Cedar Falls, the back of the car was weighed down with the books from the book sale and a couple boxes of educational items from the garage sale. As we headed home, I breathed a silent prayer of thanks for a husband who not only tolerated, but encouraged my eccentricities.

Just as joining Curves heralded a change in my attitude towards the importance of taking care of my own self, our night away signified a tremendous change had taken place in our relationship. Before cancer entered our lives, I'm convinced I would not have considered going somewhere alone with David or spending that much money on something as "frivolous" as a fancy hotel room. With our natural frugal natures, I knew we probably wouldn't make it an annual event, but I also knew we would continue to find ways to cultivate our marriage.

Out of the Cocoon

Chapter Twelve

Grow old along with me. The best is yet to be.

—**Robert Browning**

In the ensuing months, David's doctor appointments became our cherished "date day," when we would arrange for one of the older children to watch Abby. After the doctor's visit or a CT scan, we'd spend several hours alone, shopping or eating lunch in Dubuque. With CT scans initially scheduled every three months and three different doctors to see, we were ensured regular dates. Time alone as a couple was still hard to come by, considering there were several children and varying bedtimes to deal with, but we discovered my early morning wakeup time was good for more than just writing.

The children sometimes asked why their Dad slept in my office instead of with me in our bed after his cancer treatment. At first glance, our unorthodox sleeping arrangements belied our new resolve to be near each other at all times and to treat each other with respect and love.

After his surgery and treatments, David had very little saliva and his mouth was always dry. He coughed a lot at night, and because he sipped water constantly, he got up several times a night to go to the bathroom. In deference to my need for uninterrupted sleep, he chose to sleep on a mattress in my office. The difference in this "displacement" was that it was his idea and we utilized this choice to improve our relationship. We hadn't felt it necessary to explain to the kids that with my early morning rising time and Abby still climbing into my bed at night, David's sleeping in another room actually meant a ten-fold increase in opportunities for intimacy.

David would lay down by me and Abby every night holding her hand, something she requested after he came home from the hospital. Once she was asleep, I transferred her to her own bed. David and I would often remain on the big bed, just holding each other. If he didn't fall asleep with me, we'd kiss each other good night and he'd go downstairs to sleep, where I'd often join him early the next morning. This musical-bed arrangement worked for us for a year, until we moved in early 2008.

Truly heralding a new life after cancer, we bought our first house in February 2008 at the ages of forty-eight and fifty-six. That winter would be one of the harshest on record for Iowa, and we looked forward to leaving the cold farmhouse behind. Despite spending over two thousand dollars on heating bills the winter before, the house was never warm.

We weren't getting any younger, and living out in the country was becoming too difficult for us, especially since David could no longer tolerate extreme temperatures. Shortly before Thanksgiving 2007, we'd made the decision to move. Around the same time, I read a newspaper article about a first-time homebuyer's program where qualified buyers weren't required to provide a down payment. By mid-December, we were approved and began searching for a house in Manchester, where David continued to work at a nursing home.

The only regret I had about leaving the old house was all the effort I had put into decorating the kitchen and the downstairs bathroom. It had taken me years of garage sale finds to decorate my apple kitchen and a rose-themed bathroom. I'd even joked with our daughter Elizabeth that I needed to find a house with both those features.

The very first house the realtor showed us was a four-bedroom within walking distance of our oldest daughter and son, the park, the library, and even David's workplace if necessary. I loved it the minute we stepped into the foyer and spied the old woodwork. I was thrilled to discover it had an apple-themed kitchen, and then momentarily disappointed when the downstairs bathroom didn't sport roses on the wall. But then I felt a distinct shiver at the back of my neck when the upstairs bathroom revealed a delicate rose pattern on the wallpaper. God couldn't have been any more obvious that this was the house meant for us. It was like coming home.

While we continued to look at other houses in our price range, I knew we'd already found our home. We put in an offer on the last day of the year and the next day received word from the realtor that our offer had been accepted.

I immediately began the overwhelming task of cleaning and organizing for what we knew would be our last move ever. I couldn't do much else by then, anyway, due to a continual onslaught of snow and ice. I was basically stranded out in the country. By mid-February, nearby farmers had dug out a narrow, one-lane path on the road past our house, but county plows hadn't been by for days. Unprecedented in the ten years we'd lived there, mail delivery was suspended for a week because of the difficult driving conditions. Dan loaned David his four-wheel drive vehicle just so he could get to work. I was stuck inside with the children and thought I might go stark raving mad with cabin fever. Instead, I concentrated on sorting through massive quantities of books, papers, art paraphernalia, and junk we'd accumulated since our last move.

On April 19, after we'd loaded up the moving truck, I drove our van down the deep muddy ruts in our driveway and looked back one last time. The old brick house looked sad and lonely, still surrounded by huge piles of snow. I felt a surge of excitement at the prospect of beginning a new life in a place that would be much more comfortable for David.

I'd never imagined what town living would be like for us, but we easily settled in, welcomed by several neighbors and family members who lived or worked nearby. Just three weeks after our move, we were handily accessible to babysit for our two grandchildren while Elizabeth gave birth to the third.

Town living had other advantages. The kids dusted off their bicycles and rode or walked to the library several days a week. My Curves membership expired, so for the majority of that summer, I met my sister Angie for daily morning walk and talk sessions.

By August of that year, we felt as though we'd lived in our new home forever. Our son Dan bought the duplex across the street to convert into a single family dwelling, and Rachel temporarily bunked in a couple of the back rooms. Michael relocated to Manchester as well, so I was within walking distance of all of my children. Without the commute to work and the extraordinarily high heating bills, we were saving an enormous amount of money. Even the electric bills were half of what we'd paid in the country with the rural electricity company.

•   •   •   •   •

While we'd been treating David's doctor appointments as dates, we'd decided to take eight-year-old Katie with us for his late August checkup. It was the first time I wouldn't be with David inside the office as Dr. Alt checked out his throat. Instead, I sat with Katie in the waiting room. After thirty minutes, I started to get nervous. When David still hadn't reappeared after forty-five minutes, I had a sick feeling in the pit of my stomach. I grabbed Katie's hand.

"Let's pray for Daddy," I said, feeling close to tears. "It never takes this long. I'm afraid something's wrong."

I held Katie's hand as we prayed silently. When I looked up, I saw a male nurse standing near the entrance to the office.

"Mary?" he asked, "Dr. Alt would like to show you something."

My heart sank.

I started to follow him, then remembering Katie, glanced back. She looked terrified. The nurse hesitated only briefly.

"She can come, too, if she wants."

Katie jumped up to join us.

When we entered the darkened room, my stomach lurched and I thought I might throw up. David's face was gray; Dr. Alt's, serious.

"Is it back?" I asked David. He just nodded.

This was our worst fear realized. I imagined I heard the unmistakable sound of the other shoe dropping.

Dr. Alt asked Katie if she would be OK while he showed me the inside of her Daddy's throat. She nodded, but I stepped in front of her while he threaded the tubes through David's nose and down his throat. And there it was: the kind of growth I recognized from our first visit to Dr. Alt's office.

"It's a suspicious growth on the epiglottis," Dr. Alt observed. "It wasn't there at the last appointment."

"Is it cancer?" I asked, pointlessly, since I knew the answer. It looked nearly identical to the tumor that had been on the back of David's tongue.

"We don't know yet. I have to do a biopsy. But I'm 99 percent certain it is cancer. If it is, I can probably do surgery through his mouth this time so it won't be as invasive. You know he can't have radiation there again because he's already had his limit in that area, but he might be facing chemotherapy along with surgery."

I mouthed "I'm sorry" to David before leaving the room with Katie while Dr. Alt attempted to remove enough tissue for a biopsy.

Out in the waiting room, I paced back and forth. I couldn't stand the thought of David going through all of that again. And I knew that if the cancer had come back before the two-year mark, David's prognosis was not good.

Katie was uncharacteristically quiet. "Is Daddy going to be OK?" she finally whispered.

"I don't know, Katie. His cancer might be back."

Later, David would tell me that when Dr. Alt found the growth and asked if his wife was in the waiting room, David had replied that yes, she was out there with our daughter. The nurse asked what our names were so he could call us back to the room. David had replied, "Mary and . . . Mary and . . . ," and then drawn a blank. He was so shocked at Dr. Alt's pronouncement that he couldn't remember which daughter was with us or what her name was.

Dr. Alt's office called the next day. The biopsy had been inconclusive because they hadn't been able to get a big enough sample. David would need a surgical biopsy under anesthesia. It was set for late September, more than a month away. I hung up the phone and then picked it right up again. What kind of advocate was I was going to be for David this time around? A persistent one, I decided. I called the office and asked if there was a way to speed up the process. The receptionist seemed flustered as she tried to explain the standard procedure: how David had to see our family doctor, papers had to be filled out, and Dr. Alt and the surgery area had to be available.

It was Wednesday, August 27.

"He can see our family doctor tomorrow and then we can come to Dubuque to fill out the papers," I said.

"But Dr. Alt would need to be available. The operating room would have to be open . . . " she persisted, caught off guard.

By now I felt like I knew what kind of doctor Dr. Alt was. He liked things to go smoothly, had no patience for dawdling or the obtuse. He was a consummate professional who thrived on early hours and timely procedures. I knew if anyone could make it happen sooner, he could.

"Then find out if Dr. Alt can perform the biopsy earlier and if there is an open spot in surgery and get back to me today. I'll call our family doctor in the meantime and set up an appointment for tomorrow."

I was taking a lot for granted by now: that Dr. Alt would even want to schedule the surgery earlier, that the surgery room would be available, and that our doctor would fit David in. I didn't care. No one should have to wait a month to find out if their cancer has returned.

The receptionist called within the hour.

"Can you be here Friday to fill out papers? Dr. Alt said he can do the biopsy next Wednesday at seven in the morning. You'd need to be here by five."

"We'll be there," I promised, then remembered to add, "Thank you. And please thank Dr. Alt."

I hung up the phone, triumphant. I could do this. We could do this. Together we would get through whatever came our way.

David's surgical biopsy was supposed to take less than an hour. After forty-five minutes, the nurse came into the waiting room and sat down next to me.

"I just wanted to let you know the biopsy will take longer than we expected. We just got the breathing tube in. Your husband has a lot of scar tissue built up inside from the previous surgery and the radiation treatment. It's in now, though, and Dr. Alt is doing the biopsy."

Later, after David had recovered sufficiently from the anesthesia, we were informed that Dr. Alt wanted to see us. Inside his office, he broke the news that if the biopsy did show cancer, he would be unable to remove the tumor through David's mouth as he had hoped. "The scar tissue has built up too much. I wouldn't be able to get both a breathing tube and the tools needed down in there. As soon as you were put under, your throat tightened up even more."

David would need the tracheotomy and an extended stay in the hospital once again. We were devastated. Dr. Alt could see that. "The only other option would be to do the procedure with you awake," he commented wryly.

"Could we do that?" David asked. I looked at him and realized he was serious. Dr. Alt looked as shocked as I was. I knew David hated the experience of the last surgery but couldn't imagine someone willing to go through that kind of pain awake!

"I hated the tracheotomy," he said vehemently.

"Remember the biopsy I did here in the office when the tissue sample turned out to be too small?" Dr. Alt asked gently. "The pain would be much worse than that. Let's just take this one step at a time. We don't even have the results of the biopsy yet. We'll probably know by Friday, and then I can talk to some specialists who use cutting-edge laser surgery to see if that would be a possibility."

"But we are pretty sure it is cancer, aren't we?" I asked again.

"Yes, but a biopsy will also tell us if it is the same kind of cancer, or not. A different cancer would actually be better because if it is the same one then that means the original cancer was so aggressive it survived the surgery, chemotherapy, radiation, and the clinical trial drug."

So the best we could hope for was that this was a different cancer than the original?

The wait was interminable. I couldn't even pray. What would I pray for? That this was a different cancer? I didn't want David to have *any* cancer. It felt awful not being able to do something as simple as praying. I didn't dare to pray for David's healing. How could I? What if the answer was no?

I confided to my friend Pam through an e-mail that I was having trouble praying. Pam had been my pen pal for fifteen years. Besides raising a large family herself, she was a strong Christian, a woman I frequently called my prayer warrior.

Her return e-mail came on Friday morning:

> *Mary,*
>
> *It helps me so much to remember God is our Heavenly Father and we try to do the best for our own children. They may ask us for a pony or a swimming pool, or whatever . . . and sometimes we have to say "no," but we have better things in mind for them.*
>
> *Besides, you're asking for David, not yourself, and it certainly isn't wrong to desire health for your beloved.*
>
> *Dear Lord, I pray that you will show your heart to Mary for her dear husband, David. Give Mary peace as she relies on your love for her and David. You are always Our Healer, Lord, and we truly trust in your ability to inspire and direct the medical people around David . . .*
>
> *Thank you, Lord, for your Holy Spirit who helps us pray, even when we do not have the words. Honor Mary and David's generosity because they have laid down their lives for each other and their family and have inspired so many to trust in You.*

Mary and I pray together that your will be done on Earth for David as it is in Heaven, where you have said there is neither sickness nor sorrow. We speak perfect health to David, in Jesus' name.

Amen.

I read her prayer out loud and it unleashed fresh tears. This was what I wanted to pray, what I didn't dare pray for. I vowed right then that whatever the outcome of the biopsy, I would be there for David. And I would be strong, for his sake.

By late afternoon, I still waited for a call from Dr. Alt's office. Dan stopped to see how I was holding up. I told him about my friend's e-mail that morning and how I'd been scared to pray before that.

"What would you do if you found out it wasn't cancer?" he asked.

"I can't even hope for that. Dr. Alt is so sure. It looked just like the cancer on his tongue. I don't even want to have false hope like that."

"But what would you do?" he persisted. "I just want to know."

"I'd run out in the street and kiss the first stranger I saw, I'd be that happy."

Dan laughed.

By 5:00 that afternoon, I'd given up hope. We'd have to wait until after the long weekend to get the news. When the phone rang just a few minutes later, I headed down the basement steps, phone in hand. I didn't want the kids to see my reaction to the bad news.

"Mrs. Kenyon?" the nurse on the other end asked.

"Yes?" I gripped the phone tightly, waiting.

"We got back the results of your husband's biopsy. Dr. Alt wanted me to call you." Then she paused. "It was negative. It isn't cancer."

I gasped in surprise. "What? It isn't cancer? Are you sure? Dr. Alt was so certain it was cancer."

"The results were conclusive. The growth isn't cancer. Dr. Alt thinks it must be an ulcer of some sort formed from your husband's continual coughing. He'll want to see David in his office in two weeks to check on the healing of the biopsy site." She told me a date and time, and I concurred. Later, I would have to call the office to check on the appointment since I had pretty much stopped listening after the "it wasn't cancer" part.

I ran up the basement steps and out the front door, and stopped. The street was empty. The sun shone brighter. The air was cooler. My feet felt lighter. I felt as though I could have floated across the street, but instead, I ran. Dan met me at his door.

"What's wrong? Why are you running?" he asked.

"There are no strangers in the street!" The concern on his face changed to disbelief, then joy. His huge smile matched my own.

"It isn't cancer?" he asked, and we both laughed in delirious relief.

That evening, when David got home, all of us waited on the porch. He got out of his car, walked around to the passenger side, and leaned in to pull out a vase of beautiful flowers. He came up to the porch and presented them to me.

"I talked to the Human Resource Director today about getting time off for surgery, and she said her husband had given her these for her birthday. She told me to give them to you because right now you needed them more than she did."

I reached out, touching his chest lightly. "Well, you can give them back to her tomorrow. The biopsy results came in. It wasn't cancer."

"Are you kidding me?" I would never forget the wide-eyed look on his face and the broad smile that followed. It isn't every day a person wins the lottery, and that is what had just happened to us.

I knew we would never take David's health for granted again. The fear of a recurrence would likely be with us forever, but at least for the moment we knew David was fine.

•   •   •   •

Now that we felt more confident about David's health, it was time I started considering my own health. I scheduled my first baseline mammogram in October but then was called back for a repeat procedure. When those results were deemed suspicious, our doctor's office set up a consultation with a surgeon who was fairly new to the practice.

"Look at all these areas of calcification," he said as he pointed out the little white dots on the films.

"We need to do a biopsy from each breast, and if more than one of those is positive for cancer, then it would probably be best to just lop them off."

Lop them off? I couldn't believe what I was hearing and from the ashen look of my husband's face, I knew he couldn't either. For a second, I was more worried about David than myself.

"My husband only recently completed cancer treatment," I said in a warning tone, motioning towards David.

The surgeon hastened to add, "It likely isn't cancer, but if it is and that many areas were affected, it would be best to do a complete mastectomy."

"Could those areas of calcification be due to my extended years of breastfeeding?" I asked.

"I don't know. I don't think so, but don't worry. It probably isn't cancer. I'd like to do a core biopsy from each breast and we'll go from there."

I got on the computer as soon as I was home, searching for information on calcifications and worrying over the likelihood that calcifications could mean cancer. When I googled "calcifications in post-lactating breasts" my search only produced four hits, while "breast calcifications" had produced closer to four *hundred thousand* results. Evidently, there had been little research done on the difference in post-lactating breasts. The one study cited was conducted on only four women who were at a high risk for breast cancer and had a mammogram either while still breastfeeding or shortly after weaning. Of those four, all had numerous areas of calcification, but only one was eventually diagnosed with cancer.

I was amazed that this subject wasn't more thoroughly researched, especially with the increasing number of women who postponed childbirth until after the age recommended for their first mammogram. Surely there was a difference in breasts of post-lactating women that should be addressed in the medical community. Wouldn't many women be undergoing unnecessary and painful biopsies otherwise?

These were questions I wanted to ask the surgeon before having a biopsy, but not the same surgeon who had so cavalierly mentioned "lopping off" my breasts. If I had learned nothing else from David's cancer experience, I knew to be an active participant in my medical care.

The nurse seemed very disappointed when I called to cancel my biopsy with the surgeon and requested an appointment with an older, more experienced doctor. "He needs to perform ten biopsies to get his official certification," she explained about the doctor who had so casually mentioned the removal of my breasts, but this explanation only served to convince me I was not going to be one of the ten. She hastened to transfer me to the older doctor's nurse when I mentioned that the "lopping off my breasts" comment had triggered my decision.

At my next appointment, the veteran surgeon clipped the films to the overhead light and stood for several moments, arms crossed, studying them. He turned to me then, and using his pen, pointed out spot after spot, then rested the pen on two distinctly clustered areas, one on each breast.

"I have never seen so many calcifications in one woman's breasts," he stated.

"Have you ever seen a mammogram of a woman's breasts that have nursed eight children for a total of almost eighteen years?" I countered.

"No. And I'm wondering if that has something to do with it. I don't think this is cancer. I'll be surprised if it is, but I'd like to do a surgical biopsy on each breast, just in case. If those biopsies are negative, I'd feel comfortable taking a wait-and-see approach on the other areas and doing a repeat mammogram in three months."

That seemed reasonable, and the biopsies could put both our minds at rest. I could endure a little pain and discomfort for peace of mind. While I had granted permission for the initial doctor to be in the room while the biopsy was performed, no one seemed to think it was necessary to ask me if he could perform one of them. When the second biopsy was hurting much more than the first, I looked up to the see the veteran surgeon standing at my head, which meant the other doctor was sneaking in his needed hands-on experience. Lying face down on a table with my breast fully exposed and vulnerable to pokes from a large needle, I was in no position to complain. I remained quiet, but inside, I was seething.

My fury was tempered by the fact that both biopsies turned out negative. Three months later, at the repeat mammogram, all the calcifications were gone. I could have avoided the whole cancer scare if I'd only waited longer for my initial mammogram. My only regret would be that I never complained about the mid-procedure doctor switch. While I'd become an advocate for David during his cancer treatment, I hadn't yet learned to become my own.

The long past-due mammogram wasn't my only health concern. I ended up having gallbladder removal surgery and a hernia repair in late October as well. In an effort to advocate for myself, I even allowed for the luxury of staying overnight at the hospital when the doctor suggested my level of pain warranted overnight observation. Previously, I would have felt too guilty to leave my children to do so.

Months after our move, Katie and Abby were invited to jump on the neighbor's trampoline, a trampoline we'd declared off-limits when we'd moved in. They were unaware their dad watched from the window. He told me later that they'd looked around stealthily before climbing up on it and wildly bouncing. Both of them had gotten down by the time David came out of the house. But when five-year-old Abby saw him approaching, she glanced back at the trampoline with heartfelt longing and then scrambled up the side to get in a few more manic bounces before he grabbed her.

I knew just how she felt. Her dad and I were excited about the rest of our life together. We wanted to get in a few more bounces. We looked forward to watching our children grow up, to seeing our other children marry, and to holding more grandbabies. We wanted to travel together someday, and maybe even ride an airplane. "Grow old along with me. The best is yet to be," became our new motto.

Unfortunately, that was not to be. The "rest of our life together" would be just five and a half years post-cancer.

Chapter Thirteen

Epilogue: The Final Chapter

Music I heard with you was more than music, and bread I broke with you was more than bread.

—Madeleine L'Engle,
Two-Part Invention

"I wish everyone could have what we have." David took my hand across the kitchen table. I squeezed his in response.

"Do you think we could have gotten our relationship to this point without the experience of cancer? Or do you think we were so bogged down in the realities of everyday life that we would have gone on that way for years, until one day all the children would be gone, and we'd stare at each other and not have anything to say?" I asked.

By March 2012, David and I had come full circle. Reminiscent of our dating days, we now had time to sit and talk for hours, holding hands and drinking copious amounts of coffee. Twenty months before, due to a decline in both his strength and his general health, David had lost his job in maintenance and was home full-time.

Initially, when David realized that his supervisor and the Human Resource director at the nursing home were carefully orchestrating his dismissal, his intention was to fight it every step of the way, with me at his side in the role as the supportive wife. We hired a lawyer, and David followed her good advice not to quit his job prematurely. Yet the writing was on the wall: David was going to lose his job. One of the after-effects of David's chemotherapy seemed to be increased confusion, particularly with the double-speak his superiors were employing in increasingly frequent meetings. Once he realized their intention, he began requesting that I be present in the room during private meetings with the HR director and his supervisor. He was not being paranoid; it was obvious after the first meeting I attended with him that their ultimate goal was to get David to quit his job. They'd pulled out the big guns in encouraging him to leave on his own, insisting that he would soon be required to fulfill portions of his original job description which would require tasks that were well beyond his post-cancer capabilities, tasks he'd never been required to perform before cancer treatment.

"They can do that," the lawyer warned. We were simultaneously saddened and angered by the subterfuge that went on behind closed doors in an effort to force David to leave.

"Don't take it personally. It's just a business decision," the lawyer consoled him, but my husband couldn't help but be hurt.

David had asked permission for me to accompany him at that final meeting. Despite my misgivings at the prospect of observing my husband being fired from his job, I acquiesced. If David wanted me present, I intended to be there. I could barely suppress the anger I felt toward staff members who had been less than honest with him in the previous weeks. When I pointed out an inconsistency in a superior's recent actions, the room went quiet. No explanation was forthcoming, but it didn't really matter at that point. Having an advocate speaking in his defense had made a difference for David. He was able to walk out of the workplace with his pride and dignity intact. A year later, missing some of his co-workers and residents, he would offer to do volunteer work at the same place of business that had fired him.

After observing David those first weeks at home, I no longer wondered why his superiors had felt the need to let him go. Instead, I marveled that he had held on to his position for nearly four years after his cancer. The treatment had aged him drastically and affected him in a myriad of ways: from atrophied muscles in his shoulder area, to "brain fog," dizzy spells, and a generalized weakness and continued fatigue. Why had no one felt the need to warn us that the treatment itself could have detrimental side effects on David's body? Even more surprising was that I hadn't noticed the dramatic decline in his physical stamina and strength.

Initially, it would seem the worst thing that could happen to a cancer survivor, but the job loss turned out to be a blessing in disguise. I was grateful David no longer had to struggle to get through long workdays. Eventually, he qualified for disability. Having another parent at home meant that when my mother was diagnosed with terminal cancer in August 2010, I could be there for her. David was home with the kids during the week that I stayed with her while she lay dying. She died on November 3, on my fifty-first birthday.

Less than six weeks later, I could freely accompany our oldest daughter, Elizabeth, to the hospital where her five-year-old son would be treated for a Wilm's tumor. Yes, the looming specter of those cancer statistics we'd unearthed in 2006 had become a dismal reality for our family. I could only remember seeing David cry twice in our life together, including that episode of sobbing I'd interrupted in the bathroom after he'd completed his cancer treatment.

The third time I saw my husband cry was the morning I informed him our grandson, Jacob, had cancer.

Jacob immediately underwent surgery to remove a kidney and the surrounding tumor. He spent the week of Christmas in the University of Iowa children's hospital, and my daughter Elizabeth stayed with him for nearly two weeks as he recovered. Jacob would also undergo radiation and chemotherapy in an effort to eradicate the cancer that had spread to his lungs and abdomen area. He was declared cancer free in August 2011.

Seven months later, in March 2012, I was babysitting for my other two grandchildren when Elizabeth and Ben called from the hospital where they'd taken Jacob for a follow-up CT scan. David was standing on the porch when I returned home. He wrapped his arms around me as I cried into his chest. "Jacob's cancer is back," I managed to choke out.

"I know," he hoarsely whispered back.

Then my husband disappeared to the backyard for the rest of the afternoon to rake leaves while I went inside the house. That evening, David's shoulder ached horribly. Since he'd often had pain associated with vigorous physical activity, we assumed it was from the raking he'd done, and treated it with ibuprofen.

A few nights later, I was shaken awake by a cold, clammy hand. David stood at the side of the bed, swaying a little. "The pain is much worse. I feel like I'm dying. I'm cold, then hot, and I feel dizzy and nauseated." He shakily lay down next to me.

"Should I take you to the hospital?" I asked, but we both hesitated at the suggestion since he'd just lost his insurance days before. He'd experienced similar episodes in the years since his cancer treatment, usually before or after a fainting spell. I went to the bathroom and returned with a cool washcloth. David visibly relaxed as I washed his face and neck. "I'm feeling better," he sighed as his eyes closed. He fell asleep clutching my hand.

The next morning I noted the bottles of pain reliever on the table and pills scattered around the floor. Realizing just how intense his pain must have been, I called the doctor's office.

"Are you having any trouble breathing? Does your chest hurt at all?" our doctor asked as he examined him, and David shook his head. We all agreed that the marathon raking session days before was likely responsible for the intense shoulder pain. After all, while it seemed to be more intense than usual, this pain was familiar to David. "Let us know if anything changes," Deb, our favorite nurse, warned as we left the office with a new prescription for stronger pain medication.

Something changed. Two mornings later, I found David already up in his recliner when I came downstairs, his hand splayed across his chest. "I think the pain has moved to my chest. When I breathe in and out, it hurts more," he elaborated, and this time I didn't hesitate.

"You need to take him to the emergency room," the reception-ist told me when I called the doctor's office. David and I joked all the way to the hospital, certain that we would be informed he was having a bad reaction to the new medication. I'd tucked some cash into my purse, hoping to get a discount on the emergency room visit. Within minutes of our arrival, I knew the amount of cash I'd brought wouldn't even begin to cover the costs for a visit that now entailed a heart monitor, blood tests, oxygen, IV, and the nitroglyc-erin pills that were being administered under David's tongue.

"You've had a heart attack, or are having a heart attack," the doctor informed my husband. "We need to get you to the Dubuque hospital." David's eyes widened in disbelief. Everything seemed to be happening in slow motion from that point on: watching David being loaded into an ambulance, calling our son Dan to come drive me to the hospital, the interminable wait for him to get to me, our mutual stunned silence as I got into his car, then our conversation peppered with questions as we sped to the hospital, and finally, the all-too-familiar time shared in a hospital waiting room before a heart surgeon met with us.

"I've just performed a stent surgery on David. It was a bad heart attack, or a series of smaller ones." The surgeon nodded his head as we related David's recent shoulder pain, along with the bouts of dizziness, cold sweats and nausea. "He was likely experiencing a heart attack then," we were informed, and my son's eyes met mine in mutual anguish for not having seen the obvious.

Later, as I attempted to lean over the high sides of the hospital bed to kiss David, I couldn't reach either his forehead or his lips, so I began kissing the length of his arm.

"I love you," I told him before I was ready to leave for the night.

His beautiful brown eyes locked with mine.

"Thank you," he replied simply, grabbing hold of my hand with his. I brought it to my lips in response.

Thank you, as if my love were a great gift to him, when all along his love was the gift to me.

I brought David home on a Friday, nine days after his surgery. That following Monday he was to see our family physician. As David shuffled to the van like an old man, he held onto my arm for support. "I'm sorry I'm so slow," he apologized, and tears of tenderness sprang to my eyes.

It occurred to me as I buckled the seat belt around him that his health might not improve dramatically and this may be our marriage relationship from that point on: him leaning on me. My resolve to always be there for him was strengthened. "It's OK," I consoled him. "Just give yourself some time. You'll get stronger."

"His legs are still so swollen," I pointed out inside the office, and Dr. Tomas examined them carefully. The nurses and doctor at the hospital had dismissed my concerns when David was being discharged. "Those are not my husband's legs," I'd informed them incredulously. When they responded that his legs looked fine, I reminded them I'd lived with the man for over thirty years and that he was nearly fifteen pounds heavier then when he came in. They dismissed that observation as well.

"His legs are getting better. He did lose six pounds over the weekend," I acknowledged, suspecting that the extra fluid could be from the IV. I remembered being unable to tie my shoes after my surgeries because my feet had been so swollen.

"I can't see your heart, but it looks like you are healing well," the doctor concluded the visit. We would be seeing the heart surgeon for a follow-up appointment that Friday.

On the way home, David leaned back in the passenger seat, glancing over at me as I drove. "Why would God allow a little boy to get cancer?" he asked quietly, and I just shook my head in response.

"If I could go, and Jacob could stay, I'd go in a minute."

"I know you would," I whispered hoarsely as I patted his leg. The ramifications of his declaration were too painful to ponder. David would die for that little boy he loved, I had no doubt, just as he would give his life for me or for any one of his children. That was the kind of person he was. I grabbed hold of his hand, and we rode in silence the rest of the way home.

The next morning when I came downstairs, David was in his recliner, his eyes closed, looking as though he'd fallen asleep with the television on. I went out to the kitchen to make coffee, and then sat down on the couch to write. Half an hour later, I stood over my husband to wake him, gently shaking his arm.

He didn't respond. I froze. Then I shook his arm harder, calling out his name in an anguished voice I didn't recognize. "No," a moan escaped me before I ran to the phone and dialed 9-1-1.

Sometime during the night, my husband's heart had stopped beating, and I was certain that mine would break in two. It had taken years of marriage and a bout with cancer, but we'd finally discovered the joy of a good relationship. David had loved me completely, and I had learned what it was to truly love him in return.

And now?

Now, I had to learn how to live without him.

Chapter Fourteen

Reflections on the Gift of Cancer

What seems to us bitter trials are often blessings in disguise.

—Oscar Wilde

David and I had many deep conversations during the months preceding his death, conversations we wouldn't have been able to have before his cancer because he would have become impatient with my incessant need to talk things out.

"You've already talked about this. Why do you always need to rehash everything?" he used to say in an angry tone that left me cold. I'd abruptly stop talking, blinking back hurt tears.

Post-cancer, David and I talked about everything, and he would listen patiently as I dredged up some of the darker memories in an attempt to figure them out. "What had gone wrong with our marriage?" I would wonder out loud, but David never responded in anger. He knew I no longer put the blame on him. He patiently listened as I dissected everything from his hair-trigger temper to my mothering style.

I'd read all the books and the articles in nearly every magazine on the stands—those that insisted couples have a date night every week and that admonished couples not to let children come before the marriage. For years I'd shrugged that advice off, rationalizing that those articles didn't apply to me—they couldn't possibly apply to a homeschooling mother of eight children. I assumed, rightly so perhaps, that the writers had fewer children, more money, and infinitely more leisure time than we did. A weekly date would be a waste of money for a couple on a tight budget like ours, I thought, and a waste of precious time, too. I was reminded of my maternal grandmother in the hospital waiting room after my grandfather had died. It was the year before I'd gotten married.

"I wish I had treated him better," she sobbed, and I vowed right then never to treat a husband in the critical, haranguing way she had with my grandfather. Yet, had David died during his cancer surgery, my lament would have been the same.

For the majority of our marriage, I was so busy mothering babies and nursing on demand that by the end of the day, I didn't even want to be touched by David. During those sleep-deprived months when it was all I could do to get dressed by noon, reading articles about rekindling the fire or dating your husband frustrated me; it was just another chore on a huge to-do list that was never done.

Marriages can survive the ups and downs, I reasoned. And ours did. Our marriage *survived*. We weren't actively seeking a divorce or a way out. From all outward appearances, we were happy in our marriage. We still enjoyed each other's company and had good memories to share. Our marriage survived, but it wasn't thriving. The cumulative years of neglecting our relationship had resulted in a stagnant marriage. We were like so many other couples: stressed to the max and using all our energies to keep up with bills and babies. We didn't imagine that it could be any different. And it wasn't, until

David got cancer, and through our shared journey, we became part-
ners in life once again.

Initially, after David's diagnosis, I would cringe when I read
books or articles by cancer survivors who stated that cancer had
been a gift in their lives. How could all that David endured be
viewed as a gift? The invasive surgery, the weeks of chemotherapy
and radiation: a gift?

Yet, after the cancer, David would often reach for my hand and
say, "If it is cancer that is responsible for our new relationship, then
it was all worth it." And I'd reluctantly agree that cancer had been a
gift in our lives. We'd both seen the other alternative: patients and
survivors who had become bitter and angry, and neither one of us
wanted to become that.

The difference in our marriage and our relationship after cancer
was dramatic. Post-cancer, I made sure to kiss David goodbye before
he went to work. We held hands when we were out in public or alone
in the car. We sickened our children with our displays of affection
within the walls of our home. I no longer hesitated to discuss touchy
subjects with David or felt like I had to hide stressful budget situations with him.

The true test of our new partnership came several months after
David had recovered from the cancer treatment. I'd neglected to
record a bill payment in my checkbook, which resulted in several
overdraft charges before I was contacted by the bank. The charges
exceeded two hundred dollars, and there was no way I could possibly cover them. Knowing I had made a promise to share all financial
decisions with my husband, I anxiously awaited his arrival home,
my palms sweaty with nerves. I sat at the kitchen table, my stomach
in knots. David immediately noticed my worried facial expression
when he entered the house.

"What's wrong?" he asked, and I motioned for him to take a seat. He listened quietly as I explained what had happened. By the time I told him the whole sordid story, my heart was hammering in my chest, and I couldn't meet his eyes. Was he angry? Would he lash out at me like he used to? David reached across the table and gently took my hand in his. I looked up and saw only tenderness and love in his expression.

"What can I do to help?" he asked, and I burst into tears. David had become my true partner in life.

While we had developed an extraordinary relationship, we had never been extraordinary people. We were just two flawed humans who eventually discovered what it was to put the other first. Post-cancer, when I gazed into David's eyes, which I did often, I clearly saw his love for me. I saw something else, too; I could see into his very soul. David had said the same thing of some other cancer patients and survivors. "I can look into their eyes and tell they have been through something."

I knew what he meant. I'd seen it in my friend Mary's eyes the first time I saw her after she'd endured surgery and radiation for thyroid cancer. I saw it in my daughter's eyes after Jacob's cancer diagnosis. I saw it in the eyes of our new friends, Ron and Lois.

In the middle of David's treatments, Doctor Gordon introduced us to Ron and Lois, a couple who was just starting out in their journey through the same kind of cancer David had. Ron had undergone surgery and was slated to begin chemotherapy and radiation. Naturally, they had a lot of questions, and we immediately opened up to them. Cancer does that, creates a kinship between patients. My heart ached for the wife, Lois, when I saw tears welling up in her eyes as she listened to the answers to her husband's questions. Normally very reticent with strangers, I reached out to cover her hand with mine.

"I know," I said, and she nodded and gulped back tears. She knew I really did understand what she was going through.

We kept in touch with them through Ron's treatment. As David's throat got increasingly sore and his voice gravelly, he couldn't comfortably talk for any length of time so it was often me who answered Ron's questions on the phone.

"Mary, are me and David going to die?" he once asked during a phone conversation.

I paused a minute, reflecting, and then answered emphatically, "Yes. You and David are going to die."

He gasped in horror, and I quickly added, "I don't know if it will be from cancer, but you and David are going to die. We all will. We just don't live like we will."

It occurred to me then: maybe we should.

Suggested Cancer Resources

Some cancer patients will want to know everything they can about their type of cancer and suggested treatments. Others, like my husband, prefer the filtered version. I was the one spending hours on the Internet, researching oral cancer and its treatments. I was the one spending time in a chat room for oral cancer patients and survivors. Whether you are a patient or a family member, there are books and websites that address your own needs. These resources can get you started.

Books and Magazines

Alternative Medicine Magazine's Definitive Guide to Cancer,
   Second Edition, by Lise Alschuler, N.D. and Karolyn A. Gazella

> If you are interested in delving into natural and complementary methods of treating cancer, then this guide is for you. A huge volume filled with helpful information, it. A great resource for post-cancer patients in how to build up their strength and prevent cancer recurrence.

Cancer Fighters Thrive

> A quarterly magazine designed to inform and empower cancer patients and their friends and family. Integrative approach to winning the fight against cancer, includes the latest in clinical research. Articles highlight patients' courage and inspiration. Can be found at http://www. cfthrive.com.

The Chemotherapy & Radiation Therapy Survival Guide, by Judith McKay and Nancee Hirano

> The only guidebook you will need to be prepared for chemotherapy or radiation. Information, suggestions, and support to help you get through treatments. Helps the patient and the family understand chemotherapy and radiation, and gives suggestions of dealing with common side effect,s as well as ideas for getting good nutrition and support.

Coping with Cancer

> A magazine for people who have been touched by cancer. Professionals, patients, caregivers, and survivors share knowledge and experiences. Includes the latest news, FDA updates, resource lists, and interviews with celebrity cancer survivors. Can be found at http://copingmag.com.

CURE Magazine (Cancer Updates, Resources, and Education)

> Offers free subscriptions, while supplies last, to cancer patients, survivors, and caregivers.

CURE, PO Box 16657, North Hollywood, CA, 91615-
9287. See www.curetoday.com for more information.
Their website also has forums and helpful resources
listed.

Living Time: Faith and Facts to Transform Your Cancer Journey, by
Bernadine Healy

As a former director of the National Institutes of Health
and a cancer survivor, Healy has written a very informative and practical book.

Today's Caregiver

A bi-monthly magazine for and by caregivers. Free
weekly caregiver e-mail newsletter available. Can be
found at http://www.caregiver.com

*Voices of Caregiving: The Healing Companion: Stories of Courage,
Comfort, and Strength*, by The Healing Project and various
authors

Filled with the true stories of caregivers from all walks
of life. Firsthand accounts from caregivers who speak
candidly about their experience and share insights.

Websites

American Cancer Society (www.cancer.org)

A good place to start if you have questions about your
type of cancer. Valuable information, guidance, and
support helpful to cancer patients and their caregivers.

Cancer411.org

> Offers clinical cancer trial information in a searchable database. Includes cancer patient resources.

CancerCare, Inc. (www.cancercare.org)

> National nonprofit agency that offers free support, information, financial assistance, and practical help to people with cancer and their loved ones.

Family Caregiver Alliance's Family Care Navigator (www.caregiver.org)

> Offers a quick way to search for support for state, national, and private support programs.

National Cancer Institute (www.cancer.gov)

> An excellent, comprehensive site for people wanting to know more about cancer, including cancer prevention, clinical trial information, links to cancer centers, and more. Sponsors a cancer information service for patients at cis.nci.nih.gov

National Center for Complementary and Alternative Medicine (nccam.nih.gov)

National Coalition for Cancer Survivorship (www.canceradvocacy.org)

> Focuses on survivors and their families.

National Library of Medicine (www.nlm.nih.gov)

PubMed (www.pubmed.gov)

> Largest medical library in the world. PubMed provides science abstracts of the latest research worldwide.

Medline Plus (www.nlm.nih.gov/medlineplus)

> Special patient-oriented site.

www.clinicaltrials.gov

> For clinical trials.

People Living With Cancer (www.plwc.org)

> A patient information site under the American Society of Clinical Oncology (ASCO).

About the Author

MARY POTTER KENYON graduated from the University of Northern Iowa with a BA in Psychology. She is widely published in magazines, newspapers, and anthologies, including five Chicken Soup books. Her essay, "A Mother's Masterpiece" was published in the January/February 2013 issue of *Poets & Writers* magazine. Mary writes a weekly couponing column for the *Dubuque Telegraph Herald* and conducts couponing workshops for community colleges, libraries, and women's groups. She does writing workshops for community colleges, River Lights bookstore in Dubuque, Iowa, and at writer's conferences. Mary's public speaking repertoire includes the topics of couponing, writing, utilizing your talents in your everyday life, and finding hope and healing in grief.

This is Mary's second book published by Familius. *Coupon Crazy: The Science, the Savings, and the Stories Behind America's Extreme Obsession*, an ethnographic history of the cultural phenomenon of avid couponing, was published in 2013, and *Refined By Fire: A Journey of Grief and Grace* will be published in the fall of 2014. Mary lives in Manchester, Iowa, with three of her eight children.

About Familius

Welcome to a place where mothers are celebrated, not compared. Where heart is at the center of our families, and family at the center of our homes. Where boo boos are still kissed, cake beaters are still licked, and mistakes are still okay. Welcome to a place where books—and family—are beautiful. Familius: a book publisher dedicated to helping families be happy.

Visit Our Website:
www.familius.com

Our website is a different kind of place. Get inspired, read articles, discover books, watch videos, connect with our family experts, download books and apps and audiobooks, and along the way, discover how values and happy family life go together.

Join Our Family

There are lots of ways to connect with us! Subscribe to our newsletters at www.familius.com to receive uplifting daily inspiration, essays from our Pater Familius, a free ebook every month, and the first word on special discounts and Familius news.

Become an Expert

Familius authors and other established writers interested in helping families be happy are invited to join our family and contribute online content. If you have something important to say on the family, join our expert community by applying at:
www.familius.com/apply-to-become-a-familius-expert

Get Bulk Discounts

If you feel a few friends and family might benefit from what you've read, let us know and we'll be happy to provide you with quantity discounts. Simply email us at specialorders@familius.com.

Website: www.familius.com

Facebook: www.facebook.com/paterfamilius

Twitter: @familiustalk, @paterfamilius1

Pinterest: www.pinterest.com/familius

The most important work

you ever do will be within

the walls of your own home.

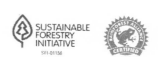

CPSIA information can be obtained at www.ICGtesting.com
Printed in the USA
BVOW04s0935150214

344910BV00004B/13/P